THE END OF DIETING
FAT LOSS FOREVER

THE END OF DIETING
FAT LOSS FOREVER

DONNA ASTON

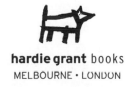

hardie grant books
MELBOURNE · LONDON

Published in 2012 by Hardie Grant Books

Hardie Grant Books (UK)
Dudley House, North Suite
34–35 Southampton Street
London WC2E 7HF
www.hardiegrant.co.uk

Hardie Grant Books (Australia)
Ground Floor, Building 1
658 Church Street
Richmond, Victoria 3121
www.hardiegrant.com.au

British Library Cataloguing-in-Publication data. A catalogue record for this book is available
from the British Library

ISBN: 9781742703695

Cover photography by Ken Pryor
Cover and text design by Peter Daniel
Typeset in Joanna 11.5/17.5pt
Printed and bound in China by 1010

ABOUT DONNA ASTON

With more than 20 years' experience, Australian-born fitness trainer and author Donna Aston has earned a reputation as an expert in the fields of weight loss, health and fitness. Having dramatically transformed her own body, Donna continues to help countless others achieve their personal goals through private consultations and training, public speaking and various publications. She has worked in Australia, Europe and the US as a private health and fitness trainer and advisor — www.donnaaston.com.

One of Australia's most sought after health and fitness experts, Donna has had guest appearances on numerous Australian lifestyle television shows. She is also a regular contributor and expert for many magazines, television and radio programs.

FOREWORD

By Dr Mei Ling Doery MBBS BMed Sci

THE TRUTH

How would you know if something were the truth? This question is foremost in my mind when I think about the mass of lifestyle advertisements, weight-loss schemes, health scams and fitness fads you might encounter on any given day. With this barrage of often conflicting information, it is more important than ever to be critical of what you read and buy into.

I first read *Fat or Fiction* as a medical student, after seeing Donna. Her approach resonated with me because it combined common sense with what science could prove about physiology. It fit with the history of industrialised food production and the current obesity epidemic. It was telling the truth.

HOW DO YOU KNOW IT'S THE TRUTH? FOUR QUICK TESTS

1. Is it contravened by other widely accepted theories (it's not a radical fad)?

2. Is it congruent with reality (no magical thinking required)?

3. Can it be seen and done in practice (can be done by a human holding down a job and social obligations)?

4. Does it stand the test of time (the person promoting it is still around after you have bought in)?

If it doesn't pass at least some, if not all, of these, look closer.

Unlike many other books peddling the answer to good health, *Fat or Fiction* did not demand magical thinking from the reader ('just believe and you will see'). And unlike the less-than-fit academics who presented the handful of nutrition lectures during my medical studies, Donna could clearly walk her talk.

Fat or Fiction passed a number of other important tests. When many were going crazy for fat-free, highly processed products and meal substitutes, Donna was teaching fundamentals and coherently arguing the case for real food.

Beyond simply providing instructions, *Fat or Fiction* delivered insight and understanding. It is this clarity above any particular piece of information that has proved most valuable to me personally and professionally, while also standing the test of time.

TEN YEARS ON

Ten years since I first read *Fat or Fiction*, there is more obesity than ever before and, paradoxically, there are many who suffer from being too thin or wanting to be. Despite great medical advances, our lifestyles are so out of shape that many of the diseases from which we now suffer are preventable. As a society we are failing to establish a sustainable relationship with our own bodies. If this trend continues, today's generation of children in the developed world is set to be the first in modern history to live *shorter lives* than their parents.

There are complex and detailed explanations for this; however, I believe the power of this book is not in its ability to analyse the problem (the medical profession is doing well at this). *The End of Dieting* is an important read because it poses the question: 'How can we be well sustainably?' In doing this, *The End of Dieting* provides a recipe for success, which is distinctly different from antifailure.

While the multibillion-pound diet industry continues to confuse and take advantage of people, setting them up for disappointment, education remains the single most powerful vaccine against the tide of preventable illness. This book is a terrific example of how motivated individuals can take charge of their health in the face of modern social and cultural obstacles. It sets forward the principles for how you can experience more than freedom from diet-induced disease, and in doing so create the opportunity to thrive.

CONTENTS

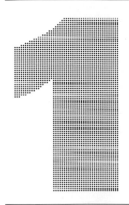
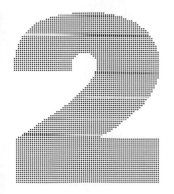

INTRODUCTION

It's now just over ten years since I wrote my first book, *Fat or Fiction*, describing how I won my own weight-loss battle and exposing how fat is not the enemy most people seem to think it is (that's sugar). But despite selling more than 120,000 copies, being joined by a host of other books (mine and other people's), and the issue being always in the media, it seems the message of how to change your body composition for the better and why low-fat (and fad) dieting is the greatest scam going simply isn't getting across. More and more clients are coming to see me totally confused. Men and women alike are so overwhelmed by complicated and conflicting information relating to fat loss, nutrition and exercise that they simply cannot see their way clear. This daily bombardment of the latest 'quick fix' to a leaner, fitter self means that the straightforward advice and solid guidance I can offer from my twenty years researching health, nutrition and exercise are needed now more than ever.

It may not be rocket science — though it is science that underpins the essential steps you need to take to transform your body and change your habits — but there's certainly an art to explaining the truth about how our bodies work. So I've developed a set of absolutely practical and essential tools (including case studies, tried-and-tested tips and tricks, and a modular menu planner) that readers can use to calculate the changes they need to make: from what exercise you need to do, and how much; to what you should eat, and when.

This is it: the instruction manual for maintaining your body that you were never given. The wait is over. In the following pages you'll find detailed explanation of the three keys to a happy, healthier you — described within the broader context of how we got to where we are, where we're all going wrong, and the future that awaits if you don't change your game.

Inspiration hasn't only come from my clients. Recently I experienced an 'aha' moment when, of all things, I was buying a new car. There I was, sitting patiently as the salesman enthusiastically thumbed through the owner's manual, keen to point out what seemed like hundreds of very foreign features, when I realised how little I really knew about what made my car 'tick'. This is how most of us feel about our own bodies. Rather than perform any maintenance, we plead ignorance and rely on some service department to deal with it. How many of us are really au fait with the intimate workings of our car's Anti-lock Braking System, Parking Distance Control or Dynamic Stability Control? Similarly, we jump blindly from one seductive diet and exercise fad to another, hoping that each will provide the answer we're looking for, because we just don't understand how it all fits together. Your car may have come with a manual (whether you read it or not is another issue) but, unfortunately, your body didn't — until now.

It's time to learn what makes you tick.

And for those of you who have some idea of how everything runs but are all too often frustrated that you don't lose weight quickly enough, this comprehensive, user-friendly 'owner's manual' will show how to make sure that every ounce of effort pays off. Yes, it does take a certain amount of dedication to get in shape and stay that way, as does anything worth striving for — if it were easy, we wouldn't have an obesity crisis. But it is absolutely doable. Now is the time to take control of your body, your health, your weight … your life.

Over the years I've found that the vast majority of clients and readers search for the diet and exercise Holy Grail strictly for weight loss. Health generally doesn't have the same urgency, at least not at the beginning. Many would probably sacrifice a vital organ to have a smaller waist or slimmer thighs. And everyone wants tangible results yesterday! Sometimes we just don't know what we're missing in terms of good health until we begin to experience it: better energy, more strength, a positive outlook, less stress, improved self-esteem … The list goes on. If you're a chronic dieter an understanding of your 'owner's manual' will reward you not only with a trimmer waistline but also the realisation that your life has been changed for good along the way.

DIET REHAB

Being an avid dog lover, I'm a huge fan of the 'Dog Whisperer', Cesar Millan, who has taken the dog world by storm. So what does this have to do with you achieving your fat-loss goals? Well, it dawned on me recently that my interest in this TV show was based on much more than my love of dogs.

Cesar's philosophy focuses on the psychological aspects of dog training. He visits dog owners and helps to diffuse problems they are having with their pets. His motto is: 'I train people and I rehabilitate dogs.' In other words, he teaches the owner to be a 'pack leader' and to understand their dog's instincts and behaviours. I see a correlation between my role and Cesar's. I train people and help them rehabilitate their bodies.

Most of us are given an unbelievably complex and resilient body to look after and maintain, yet nobody has given us the instruction manual. Consequently, over a lifetime we overfeed it with poor food choices, torture it with bouts of over-restrictive dieting, deprive it of essential nutrients, stuff it with processed carbs, neglect to take it out for regular exercise, and generally don't consider any form of maintenance until it begins to fall apart. Imagine if we treated our pets the way we treat our bodies!

So is this yet another diet book? Absolutely not. The last thing we need is another fad to lead you — along with your health, the contents of your bank account and your confidence in what you know is right — further into the dieting abyss.

This is the 'owner's manual' we didn't get. The information in this book is crucial for anyone who owns a body. Rather than a diet book, it's more like the anti-diet book. Think of it as an unbiased education on how to rehabilitate your body (and mind) and take control of your weight and your health.

Just call me the 'Diet Whisperer'!

1

WHERE ARE WE GOING WRONG?

IF THERE WERE ONLY 100 PEOPLE IN THE UNITED KINGDOM ...

81 would be adults **50** of these adults would be overweight or obese **25** of them would not be sufficiently active to improve their health **9** would use the gym **49** adults would have high cholesterol **20** adults would have tried to lose weight in the past twelve months, and only seven would believe they'd been successful **26** adults would have high blood pressure **18** adults would smoke cigarettes **19** adults would be in the 'high risk' category for weight-associated health problems **75** adults would have at least **1** modifiable risk factor for heart disease **26** adults would drink alcohol at levels considered harmful to their health **4** adults would have been dignosed with diabetes while many more would remain undiagnosed **19** would be children and **5** of them would be overweight or obese **4** children would be consumimg the recommended five portions of fruit and vegetables daily **4** adults would be affected by an eating disorder.

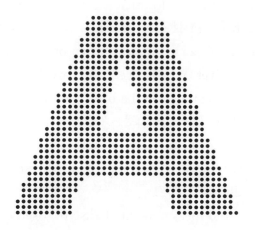

HOW DIETS ARE MAKING US FAT

MANY DIETS MAKE YOU LOSE LEAN MUSCLE AND **SLOW YOUR METABOLISM**

Most of you are likely thrilled whenever you see the number on the bathroom scales go down. But if I told you that you were potentially losing valuable muscle, you would (or should) be horrified. We only want to lose body fat.

The term 'body composition' refers to what your body weight is composed of: stored fat and lean mass. Lean mass is everything other than fat, such as muscle, internal organs and bones.

Whether you need to 'lose weight' is not related to whether you can fit into smaller jeans or whether you fit the pigeonhole of the correct height-to-weight scale but rather the fat percentage of your total weight. A healthy level for men is between 10–19 per cent. For women, a level between 18–28 per cent is considered healthy. Keep in mind it is possible (and common) to go on over-restrictive diets and become lighter yet fatter. For years we have been conditioned to pay attention to the number on the bathroom scales, full stop. How many people do you know who don't own a set of scales or don't know how much they do, or should, weigh? And I'll bet that most people (particularly women) give their bathroom scales a thorough weekly, if not daily, workout!

Most statistics and measurement charts are based on the height-to-weight scale, or body mass index (BMI). How much you weigh is somewhat irrelevant to your body's health, tone, shape and appearance due to one important but overlooked factor — body composition. According to BMI, many athletes would be falsely placed in the obese category due to their high lean-to-fat ratio, which makes them heavier on the scales.

Whether your goal is to lose fat, tone muscle, gain muscle size or become smaller, firstly you must measure your current body composition in order to set realistic goals to change and monitor your progress. This can be simply and quickly achieved with one of several types of measuring devices, some more accurate than others. Most reputable fitness trainers and sports medicine clinics can advise you on this procedure. Alternatively, you can calculate a pretty accurate figure from the formulas that follow in later chapters. From this you can determine your personal calorie requirements and accurately predict the changes you need to make to achieve your goal.

LOSE FAT, NOT WEIGHT

I have seen many men and women who could only be described as skinny. They usually do not wish to lose weight but to 'tone up'. The fascinating thing about body composition is that even if a person appears to be very thin, he or she can still have a relatively high level of body fat, therefore appearing emaciated but also soft and flabby — hence the apt term 'skinny fat'. This is caused by a low level of lean tissue and a higher level of stored body fat. The program for such people to tone up is basically the same as for a person who is overweight: reduce body fat and gain lean tissue. This is the definition of tone: high lean mass and low body fat.

For women to appear 'toned and firm', they need to achieve a body composition of around 18–24 per cent fat. For men, it's more like 10–16 per cent. Unfortunately, a lack of awareness or understanding of body composition can lead to the development of eating disorders and body-image distortions. We attempt to lose weight on the scales without realising that our real desire is to change our body composition or 'tighten and tone'. It's not just about weighing less.

Obviously appearance should not be our sole reason for improving our body composition. Health and wellbeing should be among our top priorities. By maintaining a body composition in a healthy range we can eliminate the risk of many debilitating ailments, diseases and stresses that our bodies may endure if we are overfat.

The term 'basal metabolic rate' (BMR; also known as resting metabolic rate or RMR) refers to the amount of calories the body uses in a state of complete rest (without activity) to keep us alive. Even when completely rested, the body must be burning calories at a steady rate to perform vital functions, such as repair and cell replacement, organ functions and core temperature maintenance. The BMR is determined largely by the lean weight of an individual, along with the influences of hormones, genetics and overall activity levels. The higher your lean weight, the larger your body's engine and the more fuel it will burn. Therefore more calories can be consumed before an excess is stored in the form of body fat.

An effective analogy would be to compare a large car with a V8 engine with a small four-cylinder car. If you monitor the petrol gauge, which one would burn the most fuel, even while idling? Obviously the larger engine.

As a rough estimate, for every kilogram of lean muscle tissue you gain, you will burn approximately 35 *extra* calories (or around 150 kJ) at rest. This works both ways. For every kilogram of lean muscle tissue you *lose*, whether through lack of essential nutrients or lack of physical activity, you will burn approximately 35 *fewer* calories per day. You can now see that a 'low metabolic rate', which is commonly used as an excuse for being overfat, is far more in your control than you first thought.

Statistically, the 'ideal' healthy female has around 24 per cent body fat; however, many women have well in excess of 35 per cent. Usually only elite female athletes are measured at below 15 per cent body fat. Statistically, the 'ideal' healthy male has around 15 per cent body fat; however, it is not unusual for inactive men to measure at well over 30 per cent body fat. Elite male athletes may measure at as low as 4 per cent body fat at their peak.

It's common for dieters to restrict calorie intake below the level of our BMR (our minimum requirement) in order to lose weight on the scales. What they don't consider is that the body has a very primitive yet sophisticated self-preservation mechanism designed to safeguard life at all costs. Your body doesn't know that you're intentionally depriving it of food. For all it knows, you could be stranded up a tree with no food in sight.

If you sustain this 'willpower' for long enough, your body will automatically shift gears and enter survival mode. During times of famine the body will become as energy efficient as it has to. So what does it discard first? Expendable lean tissue. This will create a smaller furnace, therefore lowering the body's BMR and hence its calorie requirements. After several weeks on this diet, like the overwhelming majority of dieters, you quit. It's just too hard to maintain so you return to your previous way of eating. But now you have lost valuable lean muscle tissue and no longer need as many calories as before, so you will store excess fat even faster and won't know why. You will eventually diet again and the yo-yo cycle will continue. And you will get fatter.

After the age of twenty-five, without regular weight-training exercise we lose an average of 200 grams of muscle tissue per year.

FAT **DISTRIBUTION**

Most of us could describe our body shape as resembling a pear or an apple. In other words, a majority of fat is accumulated either on the upper (apple) or lower (pear) section of the body.

Upper body and abdominal obesity can be quite detrimental to our health because it is often primarily *visceral fat* (within the abdominal cavity). This type of fat is more metabolically active and is much easier to shed than subcutaneous fat (directly beneath the skin); however, if an excess surrounds the internal organs it will create a strain on their functions. Abdominal fat drains directly to the liver, and can interfere with HDL (good cholesterol) production.

Although we may not like the look of it, subcutaneous fat, which makes up much of the fat on the hips, bottom and thighs, does not carry as great a health risk as visceral fat. Different concentrations of each type of fat vary between individuals.

The volume that we store of both fats is determined by our lifestyle, hormones and genetics. The stored fat in women's thighs fulfils the biological function of a reserve energy supply in the case of famine during pregnancy. This is why many underweight, malnourished women's menstrual cycles cease when body fat drops too low.

So … would you like to change your body composition and become leaner and healthier?

If the answer is yes, then read on. We're about to start work on your new body!

NATURALLY THIN?

I read an article recently about whether it's possible for someone to be 'naturally thin'. As a former fat chick who has since been accused of being naturally thin, I found this most intriguing. I have known many lean individuals who claim not to do any exercise and boast about how they eat whatever and whenever they like. While this makes many of us mere mortals green with envy, I challenge you to try keeping up with one of these people for a day. While they may not participate in intentional exercise, they usually move quickly and often. Very rarely will you find the elusive 'metabolically blessed' ones slumped on the sofa.

I have a cousin like this. Julie looks like an athlete, yet people would see her scoff a burger and fries and say, 'She's naturally thin.' I too subscribed to that way of thinking until we lived under the same roof and the 'mystery' became clear. While I'd crash out on the sofa and watch TV at night, Julie would be stretching one leg up the stairs to see how flexible she was, or obsessively vacuuming the carpet or cleaning out the kitchen cupboards. When she finally did sit down, it would last for five minutes until she was bored and would either get up and do something or start fidgeting until she drove me mad. The lesson here was obvious: she never sat still. Couple this with the fact that she never grazed or snacked on food and you have one lean chick!

Another general observation is that thin people are usually emotionally detached from food. Unlike emotional or stress eaters, they tend to lose their appetite when upset or stressed. They will often 'forget' to eat, as food is not particularly important to them. While they may eat whatever they like, they probably only eat it in relatively small quantities and don't graze between meals, therefore consuming fewer calories overall.

Ultimately, physical factors such as hormones and genetics will always play a role in our propensity to be thin or overweight, but for me lifestyle is still the most significant factor.

NATURE OR NURTURE: DO YOU HAVE THE ABILITY TO CHANGE YOUR GENES?

We've all heard the common adage 'you are what you eat', but science is now suggesting that you may also be what your grandparents ate. In fact, we now know that a person's diet can affect the next two generations.

Until recently we thought of our genes as a complex blueprint in which any evolutionary changes took place over many generations and through millions of years of natural selection. Recent studies into epigenetics may challenge this, suggesting that a single period of overeating in our youth could initiate a chain of events that would lead to grandchildren dying earlier than their peers. It seems our genes are only half of the equation. The epigenome sits above your genes and tells them to switch on or off — in other words, telling our genes how to behave. The fascinating yet frightening part of this is the evidence that our lifestyle choices can have a significant effect on the expression of our genes. Environmental factors such as diet, stress, smoking, prenatal nutrition and exposure to pesticides can make an imprint on your genes that is passed on to the next generation. Poor lifestyle decisions such as smoking or overeating can cause the genes for obesity to express themselves too strongly and genes for longevity to express themselves weakly. For example, high maternal anxiety during pregnancy is associated with the child's later development of asthma. Men who smoke in pre-puberty will be at higher risk of obesity, shortened lifespan and various health problems well into adulthood.

Those same 'bad' behaviours can predispose your children to disease and early death before they are even conceived. When our gene expression goes awry during early development the consequences may cause changes in adults that were not seen at birth. This phenomenon, called foetal programming, may play a role in many otherwise inexplicable health conditions, including heart disease, diabetes, obesity and cancer. The good news is that if you remove the environmental pressure, over time the genetic marks will fade and genes will revert to their original programming.

Our genome (hereditary information encoded into our DNA) contains all of the information needed to make us who we are, but we now know that many of the details of our behaviour and appearance are actually determined by the regulation or expression of these genes. To give you an idea of just how powerful gene regulation can be, studies have manipulated the genes of genetically identical twin mice, causing them to look entirely different in colour and size. For example, one mouse may be yellow and obese and the identical twin smaller and brown. In this case the genome remains the same, but the expression of the genes is stimulated to switch specific genes on or off. This is a great example of how 'nurture' rather than 'nature' can influence our lives.

Several environmental triggers have been shown to affect the behaviour of these genetic switches. One of these is a chemical found in many plastic drink bottles, including baby bottles, called bisphenol A. One study that exposed pregnant white mice to this chemical resulted in yellow, obese offspring (DC Dolinoy, D Huang & RL Jirtle, 'Maternal nutrient supplementation counteracts bisphenol A-induced DNA hypomethylation in early development', *Proceedings of the National Academy of Sciences of the United States of America*, 7 August 2007, 104:32, pp. 13056–061). The implications of such studies are alarming. Is there a correlation between the rise in obesity and the extensive use of bisphenol A in everything from bottles to dental sealants? Not only did this study conclude that chemical exposure during pregnancy can increase the risk of disease to an unborn child, they also observed that certain nutrients had protective properties. In particular, supplementing the mothers' diets with folic acid and vitamin B12 was shown to counteract the genetic changes caused by bisphenol A.

Many scientists are investigating how diet and other environmental stimulants influence our gene expression and disease risk. This ongoing research is likely to change our understanding of obesity and related metabolic disorders. Treatments are also being developed to silence 'bad' genes and strengthen 'good' ones. More than ever we are now aware of how much influence our lifestyle choices have over not only our health and weight, but that of our children, and their future children. Yet another great reason to look after your body, your health and … your genes!

TAKE RESPONSIBILITY **FOR** *YOUR* BODY

To control the obesity epidemic and minimise the disease risk from being overfat, we need a greater emphasis, starting from a very young age, on how best to take care of ourselves. We have responsibility for our own bodies yet it can be difficult without an instruction manual.

Experts agree that it's time to take serious action, but there is little consensus on how to tackle the global diet dilemma. There has been talk of banning poor food choices from schools and imposing a tax on and restricting advertising of junk foods.

I'm all for making healthier foods more readily available, particularly to children, but does the government really think that such negative (and juvenile) tactics of denial are a viable option? In my experience, education and support are far more productive and inspiring for people battling with their weight. Part of the problem is that we do not take enough responsibility for our bodies and our health. It is my goal to encourage individuals to take on the full responsibility for their bodies, rather than look to authorities for solutions as to how it can be collectively handled for us.

The number of diet and weight-loss alternatives available today is out of control. Meanwhile it's taken just twenty years for obesity rates to double in many Western countries, including the UK — the worst in Europe — the USA and Australia. As a result, we are at greater risk of diabetes, heart disease and a range of other debilitating ailments, which is costing billions of pounds a year in healthcare and lost productivity.

Population statistics on diet and health are based solely on weight or BMI (body mass index), which only takes into account our weight and height. In my opinion, if these statistics had been calculated using the more accurate measure of body composition (lean-to-fat ratio), the global statistics proportion of people who are overweight would likely be in excess of 85 per cent.

In our confusion and desperation we succumb to the quickest and easiest methods of weight loss. The diet industry makes millions of pounds telling us what we want to hear. Every time we pick up a magazine we are bombarded with the latest craze in how to magically melt away the fat. Needless to say, most are trying to sell us a product. Each amazing new system has a DVD, a book, a pill, recipes, a shopping guide, pre-packaged foods ... and if you call immediately, you'll receive a free gift of miracle body-shaping underwear. I am regularly frustrated by physiologically incorrect advertisements that claim you can 'dissolve' fat and shed the kilos by simply taking pills, twisting, sliding, shimmying, vibrating and (my personal favourite) 'fat zapping'.

Have you ever noticed that each new gizmo brings the promise of not only fabulous results but fabulous results *faster*? Our society craves instant gratification. Marketing gurus know that we want maximum results from minimum time and effort. I think that deep down inside we actually know the truth but we pick up the phone and give our credit card number just in case this is 'it'. While we wait for the magic solution our health is failing and quality of life diminishing. We need to take responsibility for our own body and lifestyle — today.

I recently watched a documentary about an average man who was working single-handedly to save Kakadu, a national park in the Northern Territory of Australia, from environmental threats. When asked why he was so passionate about this cause, he replied, 'I came to Kakadu and saw how beautiful it is and realised I had to do something to save it.' What set him apart from the hundreds of thousands of other people who had witnessed the same thing? Instead of walking away, he took on the responsibility.

If you blame something or someone else for the shape you're in — time, money, family, work, genetics, hormones — it will be up to something or someone else to fix it. And we all know that's never going to happen! Take responsibility for the only body you will ever have.

ONE EXTREME TO ANOTHER:
THE 'SIZE ZERO' PHENOMENON

The Duchess of Windsor's famous tongue-in-cheek comment 'You can never be too rich or too thin' brought a smile to some faces and disgust to others. While Bill Gates is doing his best to put one of these to the test, some of our Hollywood starlets may have actually cracked the 'too thin' stakes.

While the majority of women would kill to be a size eight or ten, there is currently a celebrity epidemic of the 'fashionable' US size zero. A size eight generally means no unsightly bulges; much smaller than this, however, means unsightly bulges of another kind: protruding rib cages and vertebra and bug eyes. Rumours of eating disorders are vehemently denied by Tinsel Town spokespeople, while candid paparazzi shots show minuscule party girls consuming copious cocktails and shovelling down fast food. Unlike Madonna, the majority of these women are not known for their rigorous exercise regimes and healthy diets, so what are they doing to shrink their bodies to resemble those of prepubescent children?

I've always said that if someone looks like they are starving, it's because they probably are. I've delved deeply into the phenomenon of this new breed of super-slim women and found their disturbing methods have few, if any, boundaries.

A common means of sustaining the fashionable size zero is a combination of anorexia, bulimia and substance abuse. While the pharmaceutical companies can't produce appetite suppressants and fat blockers fast enough, a growing number of prescription drugs intended to treat other conditions are becoming popular for weight loss. This is known as 'off-label' use.

One of the most common off-label drugs in the US is prescribed for the treatment of attention deficit hyperactivity disorder (ADHD).

It works on neurotransmitters in the brain to help ADHD sufferers focus on a given task. Because it is an amphetamine, it is similar to the street drug speed when taken by those without the disorder. This pill is becoming quite addictive for the modern-day party girl, enabling her to go for extended periods without food or sleep. A miracle pill, right? Wrong!

In the US these drugs are sold illegally on the street and are commonly known by dozens of slang terms. Most doctors will not prescribe these drugs for weight loss (although a minority of physicians are cashing in on the practice). Yet many desperate-to-be-thin individuals will seek these medications to lose weight. Meanwhile, we're reading the weekly gossip mags and wondering whether this is how we're supposed to look. Joan Rivers has a TV series set in Los Angeles called *How'd You Get So Rich?* Perhaps she could consider the sequel called *How'd You Get So Thin?*

My advice: stay away from all off-label drugs. Whether used alone or in weight-loss cocktails, they are potentially very risky. The majority of pharmaceuticals are powerful substances designed to correct or stabilise serious medical issues. Using ADHD medication to encourage a 'side effect' such as weight loss is like playing Russian roulette with your health. Side effects of such drugs may include sleeplessness, headaches, increased heart rate, physical and psychological dependency and psychotic episodes, to name just a few. There is a much smarter way to shed the kilos that's sustainable for the long term and doesn't put your health and your life at risk.

THE EVOLUTION OF CRAZY DIETS

Early 1900s

THE TAPEWORM DIET In the early 1900s people turned to the tapeworm as an appetite suppressant. Some tapeworm species can bring on not just weight loss, but also malnutrition, nausea, vomiting, diarrhoea, anaemia, organ damage, blocked circulation and seizures. Once in your gut, the worms have a bit of a growth spurt. So if you're okay with having a 10-metre-long scavenger in your intestines, this is the solution for you!

CHEW AND SPIT In the early 1900s American health-food faddist Horace Fletcher unveiled a new weight-loss technique. He argued that food should be chewed thirty-two times (once for each tooth) but not swallowed. The theory was that your body would absorb all the nutrients it needed and you would be able to enjoy the taste of food without the risk of weight gain. Fletcher earned the nickname 'the great masticator'. Of course, we now know that the body doesn't absorb nearly enough food through chewing alone—weight loss on this diet is due to malnourishment.

1920s

CIGARETTES Advertisements for cigarettes urged people to 'reach for a Lucky [a cigarette brand] instead of a sweet—it's better for your figure!'

1960s

THE DRINKING MAN'S DIET In 1964 Robert Cameron published *The Drinking Man's Diet*. In addition to carbohydrate control, this weight-loss book recommended that readers drink gin and vodka. The book quickly became a bestseller, but physicians of the era were up in arms (and rightly so) about the excessive amount of alcohol involved.

1980s

CABBAGE DIET This popular mid-1980s diet required followers to consume as much cabbage as they wanted for seven days (and presumably to stay away from open flames). Although recently updated to account for its lack of protein, this diet is deficient in a multitude of nutrients and obviously not sustainable.

1990s

MACROBIOTIC DIET Popularised by Gwyneth Paltrow and Madonna, the macrobiotic diet borrows from traditional Japanese cuisine, emphasising wholegrains, vegetables, beans and modest amounts of fish, and stipulates that every meal must balance yin and yang. Although it advocates a diet rich in vegetables, the macrobiotic diet can cause a number of nutritional deficiencies, including inadequate intake of protein and essential nutrients such as vitamin D, calcium and iron.

2006

BOOTYLICIOUS DIET Popularised most recently by Beyoncé Knowles, this diet requires followers to drink six to twelve glasses of lemonade laced with cayenne pepper and maple syrup. Knowles, who famously used it to slim down for her role in *Dream Girls*, was the first to concede that the diet was only a temporary fix, going on the record to say that while she did lose weight, she put it back on almost immediately after resuming normal eating. Not to mention the fact that it will likely rot your teeth and put you at risk of diabetes ...

2000s

THE COOKIE DIET This gem harks back to the mid-1970s when a Dr Sanford Siegal began recommending his 'special' cookies to patients at his Miami-based clinic. Siegal, author of *Is Your Thyroid Making You Fat?* (2001), is currently marketing his cookies from a recently opened Beverly Hills store. His anticipated revenue for the first year was US$18 million. We can't be that gullible, can we? Siegal suggests that we eat six of his special low-cal cookies per day, plus one meal, which equates to around 800–1000 calories. Not only is this diet ridiculously low in nutrients, but it perpetuates the notion that you can eat cookies for weight loss (or have your 'cake' and eat it too). These cookies cost dieters more than US$50 a week and the feedback suggests that they taste vile.

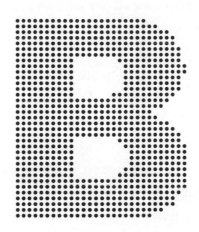

WHY THE DIET AND HEALTH INDUSTRIES AREN'T HELPING

BIG FAT MISCONCEPTIONS: WHY FAT PHOBIA IS CONTRIBUTING TO OUR EXPANDING WAISTLINES

However you look at the global obesity epidemic, the low-fat crusade has played a huge part in it. From the late 1940s, following World War II, the rate of heart disease began to rise. In the 1970s the US government issued a report advising Americans to lower their risk of heart disease by reducing the fat in their diet. This recommendation was based on evidence that linked diet to heart disease. Unfortunately the report erroneously identified saturated fat as the culprit responsible for all our health problems. This message, which soon spread around the world, was the beginning of the low-fat diet catastrophe.

Once dietary fat was seen to be the problem, the market opened wide for a surge in low-fat, processed 'faux foods' and an industry was born. Sugar and thickeners were added to foods to replace the taste and texture of fat. The race was on to engineer the saturated fat out of everything. This led to the creation of a plethora of Frankenfoods. Many decades on, faux foods such as margarine are still touted as the healthy alternative. Television advertisements feature actors wearing white coats and stethoscopes preaching the heart health benefits of chemically enhanced products laden with trans fats. So long as sugary processed foods were low fat they could even receive the Heart Foundation Tick.

Fat, the primary macronutrient that keeps you feeling full and satisfied, was now missing from most of our meals. Sugar, which keeps cravings and fat storage high, was abundant. We began to consume a higher volume of food and a greater concentration of processed carbohydrates and artificial additives. Portion sizes grew in an attempt to satiate our appetite as well as represent 'value'.

The low-fat diet may not be the only reason we're experiencing one of the worst health epidemics in history, but it has certainly played a significant part. Each of our cells is encased in a cell wall, a delicate membrane composed mainly of fats. This needs to be fluid enough to allow nutrients and information to pass through it. The food we consume has a significant effect on the health of our cell membranes. Healthy fats, such as omega-3 in fish and flaxseed, and antioxidants from colourful, fresh plant foods, will protect the integrity of our cell lining.

Too much of the wrong kind of fats, such as trans fats, can cause the cell membrane to become too rigid and obstruct the necessary nutrients from entering and nourishing our cells. Unfortunately the fats that are most prone to causing this kind of damage are the fats we're told to consume more of — unsaturated fats, such as vegetable oils. Many people assume that because these oils are derived from plants they must be better for our health. On the contrary, they are highly unstable to heat, light and oxygen and can therefore be easily damaged in extraction and processing. Regular mass-produced vegetable oils are extracted using high heat, which can make them rancid at the time they are produced. Rancid oils are highly toxic. Having gone bad, the oils are then deodorised and various chemicals are added to remove the bad smell, to give the oil a nice colour and to prevent the formation of bubbles during cooking.

Saturated fats have been the 'bad guys' for many years, yet they are actually more stable and less vulnerable to damage than vegetable oils. This doesn't mean that we should avoid vegetable oils, but we should take care to ensure they are unprocessed and that we consume them in the presence of antioxidants.

THE CALORIE **MISCONCEPTION**

Over many years of advising clients I have found that most people believe they need far more calories than they actually do. Online calorie calculators are now widely accessible, but much of the time I find their estimates of calorie requirements to be too high, particularly when we enter information about our activity to calculate calories burned over and above our minimum daily requirement, the basal metabolic rate (BMR).

In the menu planner of this book you will find an accurate BMR calculator. However, be careful not to overestimate your perceived activity. If you follow your BMR calculation honestly over a period of weeks and you do not see a significant loss in body fat, you are almost certainly overconsuming. In this case, it doesn't matter that your calculations are correct, or that it's working for your best friend. The only thing that matters is that it's not working for you, and if you continue to do the same thing you will continue to get the same result. You must either increase your daily exercise or decrease your portions by 10 per cent (or both) and you will kickstart fat loss.

Your body is a mirror image of your lifestyle. If you're 80 kilos with a goal of 60 kilos, and you get 'stuck' at 70 kilos, it's because you have the diet and exercise habits of a 70-kilo person. Tweak your lifestyle to that of a 60-kilo person and your body will have no choice but to follow you there. You might feel that you'll keel over from malnutrition if you stick to this rule of thumb, but I'm here to tell you it's actually going to be pretty close to what your body needs.

I took on a new client, Jenny, who started out at 20 kilos above her 'healthy' weight and, as a result, had been experiencing some health problems. Following an initial consultation and discussing her goals, she commenced her new regime. Two weeks later she came to my office to weigh in and discuss her progress. She was quite distressed, explaining that she would have starved to death on the amount of food I had suggested if she had kept it up for more than a day. (The plan, by the way, included three balanced main meals and two snacks each day and the appropriate amount of calories for her BMR.) I asked her what 'starving' felt like. Did she feel faint, shaky, lethargic, vague, nauseous? All of these may have indicated that she was not consuming enough food and was experiencing blood-sugar fluctuations, which we certainly want to avoid at all costs. She said her stomach felt empty, but there were no 'symptoms' as such. She felt compelled to increase the amount of food we'd recommended because she 'couldn't stand the hunger'. So I weighed Jenny and measured her body composition to compare it to her initial result two weeks prior. Not surprisingly she was exactly the same. She hadn't lost a gram of fat.

After a long conversation I started to get the feeling that much of what Jenny had experienced was a psychological attachment to food and a fear of change. Jenny left my office with a new goal — to take on the food plan with an open mind — and instructions to contact me immediately should she start feeling uncomfortable. Seven days later an ecstatic Jenny skipped out of my office having lost 1.5 kilos of pure body fat! She had experienced no hunger. In fact, she now felt she had more energy and fewer cravings. The lesson in this? Sometimes we need to let old habits die and acknowledge that change can be a bit daunting. It's a lot easier to feel full and satisfied if you focus on quality rather than quantity.

DON'T FORGET **LIQUID CALORIES**

You may be surprised to discover just how many extra kilos can creep on by overconsuming seemingly harmless beverages. Drinks are easily consumed and often not thought of in terms of calories.

- » Two standard glasses of wine each night with dinner = 1120 calories (4682 kJ) per week. Almost equivalent to an additional full day of eating every week.

- » Four 375 mL bottles of beer or three gin and tonics at a weekend barbecue = 600 calories (2508 kJ). Equivalent to one entire box of Cadbury Milk Tray chocolates or three doughnuts.

- » Three glasses of champagne = 270 calories (1128 kJ). Equivalent to a small serving of McDonald's fries or a 200-gram steak.

» A couple of creamy pre-dinner cocktails = 700 calories (2926 kJ). Equivalent to a Big Mac and four McNuggets, or three McDonald's sundaes.

» A cup of hot chocolate = 200 calories (836 kJ). Equivalent to a Classico Cornetto ice-cream or thirteen teaspoons of sugar.

So next time you're enjoying a social drink, beware of the hidden calories … or they'll be showing up in places that you're unable to hide!

FOOD **CULTURE**

We've recently witnessed the phenomenon of the TV series *MasterChef*. What a powerful machine it became, not only to propel the participants into the celebrity stratosphere, but in its overall influence and astounding marketing power. We lapped up the information on each episode. While I'm thrilled that this inspired many of us to get back to cooking at home, unfortunately it wasn't necessarily to create healthy meals. To give you an example, most retailers have had deep fryers gathering dust on the shelves for years but once *MasterChef* came along they were suddenly in hot demand.

I think somewhere along the way, between longer working hours and the increased availability of convenience foods, we've started to lose the culture of the home-cooked meal. Once a mainstay, the staple 'meat and two veg' and the preparation of 'real' food are becoming a thing of the distant past. We blame lack of time, but really I think it's lack of practice. Once you have a decent repertoire of home-cooked meals, it's easy to prepare them at a moment's notice.

WHAT ABOUT PHARMACEUTICALS FOR WEIGHT LOSS?

Despite the limited training doctors receive about the primary causes of obesity, they can be quick to prescribe medical intervention to 'cure' it. Most of us feel quite desperate by the time we admit that our weight is a problem and work up the courage to approach someone for help, and we'll try almost anything they suggest. Yet some of the most popular prescription drugs approved by authorities for the treatment of obesity are far from miracle solutions.

There are two main types of pharmaceutical interventions currently in use. The first are appetite suppressants, which are amphetamine based and alter brain chemistry. It is claimed that these drugs assist in weight loss when combined with a calorie-controlled diet and exercise (although these would provide results without the drug). Unfortunately, the outcome is generally a temporary fix, which cannot be sustained. Drugs cannot teach you to choose healthy food; they can only help you to consume less. When you stop taking them, your appetite returns to normal. Medication certainly doesn't inspire an increase in activity. As with most pharmaceutical aids, the risk of dependence is high due to fear that the weight loss cannot be sustained without the drug. There are also myriad potential side effects, including insomnia, dizziness, high blood pressure, headache, nausea and anxiety.

The other type of drug blocks fat absorption. The primary side effect of this is a leaking bowel, and it encourages a 'binge, purge' attitude to food: eat all the fat you like and it will simply pass right through you. The absorption of essential fat-soluble nutrients, namely vitamins A, D, E and K (all powerful antioxidants), is hindered by fat-blocking drugs, leading to deficiencies. Fat-blocking drugs do not discern between processed 'bad' fats and essential 'good' fats such as omega-3, and so all fats are purged, potentially causing as much damage to your overall health as obesity itself.

Yet nobody is overweight due to a pharmaceutical deficiency! While the ever-hopeful chronic dieter remains vulnerable and searching for new quick-fix fads, pills and potions, the supply will remain endless. I know that some of you will still be tempted to use drugs to lose weight, regardless of the side effects.

MY ADVICE?

» Repeat after me: There is no quick fix! There is no quick fix! There is no quick fix!

» Educate yourself to find a balance in your lifestyle for the long term.

» Prioritise your health and your food choices.

» Take a piece of paper right now and write down the single most important benefit you would gain from having a healthier, leaner body. Keep it in a prominent place and refer to it when you feel your motivation lagging.

» And finally ... just move!

BLINDING US WITH SCIENCE

The press releases announcing the results of scientific studies can sometimes be interpreted in several ways. If the media coverage of a scientific finding is confusing or contradictory, it's worth tracking down the original study to find the explanation.

Scientific research is not always as thorough or conclusive as it may seem.

» Don't eat carbohydrates after 4 pm. Why? Because a study says so.

» Don't lift weights because you will look like Arnold Schwarzenegger. Why? Because a study says so.

» Don't combine protein and carbs because you can't digest them. Why? Because a study says so.

» The first twenty minutes of exercise are almost worthless. Why? Because a study says so.

I think you're starting to get the picture. Information is crucial when managing health and I would never disparage nutritional or fitness research but there is some sense in issuing cautionary advice.

Every other day a new study comes out that sends us straight to the pantry to throw out whatever is harming us, followed by a quick trip to the supermarket to stock up on what we *should* be eating.

As the obesity crisis worsens health experts continue to surface with ever-more fantastic studies. Beware of scientific research funded by pharmaceutical companies or other interested parties, as this can have an influence on the results, or at least the angle of the press release, which is the interpretation the majority of us have access to in the news. If you go back to the studies themselves, as I do religiously, you will often find that the results have been published to favour specific products. It's possible to associate almost anything with a study if the desire is strong enough. You could feasibly suggest umbrellas cause rain as evidence indicates they are always out in a downpour!

Recently the media reported claims that vitamin C and E supplements were of no benefit to health whatsoever. Intrigued and a little surprised, I looked at the basis of the study and discovered that the experiment only used 40 mg of vitamin C, which is less than that found in a segment of orange — most supplements are either

500 or 1000 mg. It is unlikely that you would be able to find a 40 mg vitamin C supplement, as few people would be likely to take one. The researchers had also used a synthetic, poorly absorbed form of vitamin E (dl-tocopherol), not the natural form (d-tocopherol) found in foods and most supplements, rendering the vitamin virtually worthless. The study's foundation was fundamentally flawed.

One of my favourite claims is the recommendation, often issued by doctors, not to take supplements because they just create 'expensive urine'. If this were the case, you may as well give up eating and drinking too because that will create haute cuisine urine. Of course your body will eliminate what it does not absorb, but that does not mean that the nutrients in supplements are not absorbed throughout the digestive process. Urine is what is left over after your kidneys purify your blood. If your urine contains extra vitamin C, that vitamin C was in your blood. If the vitamin was in your blood, you absorbed it well. If your body excretes vitamins in your urine it's a sign that you are well nourished and have nutrients to spare, which is a good thing! 'Waste' indicates fullness, just as an overflowing petrol tank is unmistakably a full tank. Urine spillage of vitamins indicates nutritional *adequacy*, just as a lack of water-soluble vitamins in the urine indicates *inadequacy*.

William Kaufman, MD, a physician with a PhD in nutritional biochemistry, wrote: 'Those who believe that you can get all the nourishment including vitamins and minerals you need to sustain optimal health throughout life from food alone can be very smug. They have the equivalent of an orthodox religious belief: "food is everything". They don't have to concern themselves with the fact that the nutritional value of foods their patient eats may be greatly inferior to the listed nutritional values given in food tables … The two-liner "We get all the vitamins we need in our diets. Taking supplements only gives you an expensive urine" completely overlooks the benefits vitamin supplements can produce in our bodies before being excreted in our urine.'

Kaufman offers a great example to illustrate his point. 'During the early part of World War II, GIs treated with penicillin had to save all their urine so that the penicillin which had been excreted in their urine could be recovered and then used to treat other GIs with life-threatening wound infections. If one only considered the penicillin that was excreted in the urine and not the benefits that the GI had in having his infection cured by penicillin, one could sneer that penicillin's only function was to give the GI expensive urine. If one considered only the function of penicillin in the GI's body, one would have to marvel at the miracle of its curing a potentially lethal infection.' (W Kaufman, 'Nutrition illiteracy and nutritional inadequacy', *Journal of Orthomolecular Medicine*, 2007, Vol 22, No 2, pp 83–9.)

My advice is that you should take note of information that you come across in the news but don't adjust your diet and exercise until you have looked into it. Don't be blinded by science because it isn't always what it seems. Studies and experts may have an agenda or be employed by companies with a vested interest in a particular outcome. Don't let them divert you from your healthy path.

IF YOU CAN'T BEAT 'EM, **JOIN 'EM?**

The latest craze at fast-food chains seems to be offering 'healthy' options. Recognising that their faux foods are now perhaps under threat, many are making desperate attempts to become the fast-food good guys. I'm all for health initiatives, but I'm not sure the recent collaboration between a multinational weight-loss company and the world's biggest burger chain can be described this way.

In Australia and New Zealand, Weight Watchers has signed a deal with the Golden Arches to endorse some of its meals, such as Chicken McNuggets, as good choices for dieters. This is part of a six-year campaign for McDonald's to change its image. One may be forgiven for thinking that McDonald's is using its financial muscle to further exacerbate our global obesity epidemic. Why, it's even spent £215,000 to put a Heart Foundation Tick on several of its meals, including burgers and nuggets. (The fees required to become an official licensee and display the Tick are detailed on the Heart Foundation website.) It's one thing for fast-food outlets to peddle their calorie-dense convenience foods, but it's quite another for those to masquerade as healthy choices!

In this new deal, McDonald's will use the Weight Watchers logo on menu boards and tray mats, while in return Weight Watchers will promote McDonald's to dieters.

'Make no mistake, this is about selling more burgers and fries,' said Boyd Swinburn, from the Australian Society for the Study of Obesity at Deakin University. 'Mum can go in and feel good about her Weight Watchers meal while she buys the kids burgers. Anyone who thinks otherwise is naive.' The three Weight Watchers-endorsed meals include nuggets (372 calories/1560 kJ), the Filet-O-Fish (331 calories/1390 kJ) and a sweet chilli seared chicken wrap (392 calories/1640 kJ).

Government health authorities are also urging fast-food outlets to display the number of calories in a 'junk food' menu item, next to the price. While I commend the effort, it's unlikely that the vast majority of consumers (other than diehard dieters) will understand the significance of a calorie. I also have my doubts whether anyone is under the illusion that junk food is a healthy choice, so I don't believe calorie displays are likely to have much of an impact.

Sporting clubs are increasingly sourcing sponsorship from fast-food conglomerates in return for brand exposure and advertising during televised events. Some high-profile sporting personalities directly endorse specific fast-food products. If the government is going to regulate anything, surely it should be this form of advertising? Tobacco advertising has been banned from sporting events for many years now. There is a counter-argument that the money injected into sport by fast-food sponsors may encourage fans to participate in sport and exercise, but it's important to remember that obesity has surpassed smoking as one of the leading causes of disease. We cannot underestimate the influence that sporting heroes have on young, impressionable fans. If the fast-food companies were restricted to advertising only their 'healthier' options when pitching to influential sports fans, this would deliver a powerful message and might offer a positive solution for all involved.

COSTLY MISTAKES:
WHAT ABOUT THE KIDS?

Obesity rates among children are at an all-time high. The statistics are alarming: one in seven EU children is now overweight or obese, while in the US it's one in five and in Australia a staggering one in four. This life-threatening epidemic is spiralling out of control. Something must be done ... and quickly!

There are often several contributing factors to obesity, both in childhood and adulthood, including sedentary lifestyle, poor nutrition and the overconsumption of high-calorie, sugar-laden foods. Our children are now more accustomed to passive forms of entertainment, such as video games, television, DVDs and computers, as opposed to outdoor activities such as skipping rope, bike riding, playing hopscotch and rollerskating. It is generally recommended that children get around an hour of physical activity each day, but I think it's fair to say very few kids these days would get the opportunity to do this.

Parents have a significant influence on forging early behaviour. It is often the case that overfat children have overfat parents. Without a positive role model, young children certainly face a substantial challenge. Many adults are drowning in the vast sea of diets and weight-loss fads, so it's not difficult to see why their children also fall victim. Some parents lay the blame on genetics or medical conditions which are 'out of their control' when their family collectively struggles with weight gain. In reality, only 5 per cent of obese people suffer from metabolic or endocrine disorders. Laying blame on external factors is often only useful in exonerating oneself from taking responsibility — not in creating positive change.

One factor we often overlook is body composition. While we are all busily focusing on weight, we tend to ignore the important factor of how this weight is composed. A low proportion of lean muscle means a low basal metabolic rate and therefore the decreased burning of body fat and calories. This is why restrictive diets, particularly in the absence of physical activity, are ineffective for long-term fat loss.

One of the biggest mistakes a parent can make is to reduce fat and calorie intake, depriving (or essentially punishing) an overfat child. Developing bodies require optimum nourishment from food to facilitate growth and to sustain adequate lean muscle, so a sensible nutrient-rich regime is of utmost importance … including essential fats. Rather than deprivation and restriction, I suggest we try to focus on adding 'good' foods back into the diet. Educate your child on the value of nutrition and the ill effects that 'empty', low-nutrient junk food can cause to their health. I have found that getting children involved in cooking is a great way to educate them about food and broaden their palates to various ingredients.

If possible, set up a veggie garden. This not only gets them excited about growing food but helps them to understand and appreciate where healthy foods come from ... and it's not from the plastic bag or wrapper to which they may have become accustomed. I must admit to being shocked when a young checkout person at the supermarket has had to ask me what a pumpkin or a passionfruit was in order for them to process the transaction. This has happened to me several times with various teenagers, who seemed confused yet intrigued about these 'foreign' items.

When it comes to our kids, the single most important factor for parents to acknowledge is that we must lead by example. To single out a child and highlight their 'problem' is not conducive to positive behavioural change. The entire family must embrace improvements to diet and activity, with mum and dad clearly leading the way. Here are some simple 'rules' that can be adopted by the household — including parents!

» No eating in front of the television. If you're hungry, you must eat at the table.

» Chew your food properly and take your time at each meal. It takes twenty to thirty minutes for your stomach to register that you are full, so eating quickly allows us to overconsume food and not realise until it's too late.

» Eliminate junk food from your kitchen. Replace biscuits, lollies, soft drinks and ice-cream with an abundance of healthy alternatives, such as fruit, cheese, yoghurt and nuts.

» Get the kids involved in food shopping, preparation and cooking. Not only is this a valuable learning experience,

> it's likely they'll begin to enjoy and value healthy, home-cooked meals.

» Make physical activity part of your family life by encouraging long walks, playing at the park, exercising the dog and bike riding.

» Educate yourself and your children about the importance of good nutrition.

With statistics showing increasing numbers of young children developing adult-onset (type 2) diabetes, high cholesterol and other degenerative diseases formerly only associated with aged adults, it's time to take some serious action against this health-threatening epidemic before it has a profound effect on you and your family. Type 2 diabetes, usually diagnosed in adults over the age of forty-five, is increasingly being diagnosed in children. In fact, type 2 diabetes has emerged as a critical health issue in overweight and obese children.

SOME TOUGH LOVE:
LIVE TO EAT OR EAT TO LIVE?

A client once told me that her recipe book collection was divided into two categories: 'Good Donna' (Aston) and 'Evil Donna' (Hay). Depending on her mood, one was associated with moderation and discipline and the latter with rebellion and reward.

The mere suggestion of discipline tends to conjure up a negative response. Therein lies the problem: we commonly indulge in poor food choices as a feel-good reward for an otherwise regimented existence, when in reality the resulting weight gain, lethargy and poor health can hardly be considered a reward.

Finding the motivation to stick to a healthy lifestyle can be the bane of our lives. When it comes to diet and exercise, we give ourselves the option of whether we 'feel like it' or not. We all possess the discipline — we apply it to so many of the areas of our lives to which we've assigned priority. You don't neglect to brush your teeth for a week because you don't feel like it, but you choose not to exercise or eat well for that very reason.

Since we were nurtured with milk as babies, we have been conditioned to feel comforted by a belly full of food. Unfortunately, the food we often find most comforting is unhealthy and is usually consumed to excess. When you have a fight with your partner, the tub of choc-chip ice-cream will likely have more appeal than a bowl of steamed greens!

Now I'm certainly not suggesting that you must adhere to a strict macrobiotic diet, but the majority of us do need to start taking more care with what we put in our mouths — after all, it's the very 'fuel' that infiltrates every living cell in our bodies. The concentration of nutrients derived from food is vital for survival, yet overly processed, nutrient-poor foods are increasingly becoming the norm.

Colourful plant foods are a primary source of essential nutrients, yet many people do not consume adequate quantities for optimum health. This is a worrying trend when you consider that the inadequate consumption of fruit and vegetables is linked to an increased risk of developing certain cancers. While it is obvious that severely underweight individuals are at risk of nutritional deficiencies, the 'empty' calories consumed in processed food means it is also possible — even common — to be overweight and undernourished. Your body is a direct reflection of your lifestyle. The resulting damage may not be immediately apparent, but the long-term effect of a nutrient-poor diet can be catastrophic.

It's all very well to say that we should eat to live, but many of us still live to eat. Our fatty, sugar-laden diets and sluggish lifestyles have doubled England's obesity rate over the past twenty-five years, which costs the nation billions of pounds per annum in associated health-care costs and lost productivity, not to mention reduced quality of life. Despite the fact that we have access to some of the world's finest produce, our culture seems to be increasingly conditioned towards the overly processed foods and oversized portions common in American society.

We store excess body fat if we consume more calories than we burn off. To put things into perspective, it would take the average person around three hours of walking to burn off the average dessert — and that's just to break even. Processed foods offer concentrated calories void of nutrition and fibre and are therefore very easy to overconsume. They also contain a plethora of artificial additives, sugar and dangerous fats.

Now before you say, 'But I don't eat processed foods', I'm not simply referring to takeaway burgers and fries. Under this umbrella are many popular gourmet choices, such as chocolate, pastries, dips, bakery items, cakes, gravies, refined vegetable oils and fried foods. The high sugar content of refined foods can cause obesity and metabolic disorders, while trans-fatty acids have been associated with a multitude of degenerative diseases.

Instead, you could be reaping the benefits of refuelling your body's cells with nutrient-dense fresh foods. Why would anyone pass up the opportunity to have boundless energy, better-quality sleep, excellent health, high self-esteem, a toned and lean body and great skin … all while enjoying healthy food?

If you truly love food and you despise the thought of eating healthily, remember that it is absolutely possible to excite your taste buds with the right ingredients. I have been doing this for years, along with dozens of my die-hard foodie clients and friends. Make a point of learning more about quality seasonal ingredients, dust off your recipe books for inspiration and you can enjoy the best of both worlds!

DISTURBING FACTS

» The average English-speaking Western population consumes approximately 57 kilograms of sugar per person, per annum. This equates to approximately nine to ten tablespoons of sugar per day, per person.

» The average 340 mL can of soft drink contains more than eleven teaspoons of sugar.

» Carbonated drinks can rob us of calcium, which helps us to burn fat.

» Sugar is an 'anti-nutrient', which depletes your body of B vitamins and various minerals and potentially increases nervous tension, anxiety and irritability.

» Excessive sugar consumption can suppress the activity of white blood cells by up to 50 per cent thirty minutes after ingestion, and this immune suppression can last for up to six hours.

» The Centre for Science in the Public Interest in Washington, DC, suggests that reducing sugar in soft drinks by one-tenth would reduce America's annual sucrose consumption by 220 million kilograms.

» Statistically, an average adult's lean mass will decline by around 3 per cent per decade and their metabolic rate will decline proportionately. Every kilogram of lost muscle results in a fall in our basal metabolic rate (BMR) of 30–50 calories.

» 7700 calories = 1 kilogram of stored body fat. The average 60-kilogram woman with a healthy body fat ratio of 25 per cent is carrying 15 kilograms of her weight in fat — enough fuel to sustain 385 hours of walking.

» It takes twenty minutes of brisk walking to burn off a skinny caffè latte without sugar.

» If you were to consume four average-sized chocolate or confectionery bars each week, this would equate to approximately 83,200 additional calories (or 10.8 kilos worth of excess stored fat) per annum.

» A study has shown that women consuming 62 per cent or more of their calories in the form of carbohydrates (predominantly sucrose and fructose) were 2.2 times more likely to develop breast cancer than those who consumed less than 52 per cent (Isabelle Romieu, Eduardo Lazcano-Ponce et al., 'Carbohydrates and the risk of breast cancer among women', *Cancer Epidemiology, Biomarkers and Prevention*, August 2004, 13, pp. 1283–89).

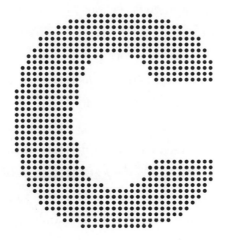

RECOGNISING THE REAL ENEMY

ARE CARBS **MAKING YOU FAT?**

A recent study published in *The Archives of Internal Medicine* (Sabina Sieri, Vittorio Krogh et al., 'Dietary glycemic load and index and risk of coronary heart disease in a large Italian cohort: The EPICOR study', *The Archives of Internal Medicine*, 2010, 170(7), pp. 640–47) has confirmed that the consumption of high-glycaemic carbohydrates increases the risk of coronary heart disease in women.

The glycaemic index (GI) is a measure of how quickly food affects your blood sugar. Those of you who have read my previous books will know that I'm not a huge fan of the GI scale, but refined carbs are generally high GI and I'm definitely a fan of decreasing all sources of them. This includes not only obviously sugary products, but also many breads, pastas, commercial cereals and white rice. Almost all vegetables and most fruits are the preferred source of carbs.

When your blood sugar rises too quickly you release a hormone called insulin into your bloodstream. Insulin takes the excess sugar from your bloodstream and directs it into storage — in other words, fat. Because these foods raise blood sugar too quickly, consuming them will almost guarantee that your body will remain in 'fat-storage mode'. This is also why I don't advocate high-carb or low-fat diets. Carbs have a significant effect on blood sugar and insulin levels, whereas protein and unrefined carbs cause only a minor response and fat has no effect at all.

If this isn't enough reason for you to cut refined carbs, a recent study (Jean A Welsh, Andrea Sharma et al., 'Caloric sweetener consumption and dyslipidemia among adults', *Journal of the American Medical Association*, 2010, 303(15), pp. 1490–97) analysed the diets of over 47,000 Italian men and women for carbohydrate intake and its impact on blood sugar. The standout result from this publication showed that the 25 per cent of women in the study group who consumed the most carbs overall (regardless of GI) had twice the risk of developing heart disease as those who consumed fewer carbs. The men and women with higher sugar consumption (>10% added) showed that low HDL (previously good cholesterol) levels were increased by as much as 50–300 per cent compared to the reference group (<5% added). In conclusion, there was a statistically significant correlation between dietary sugars and blood lipid (fat) levels — a profile associated with cardiovascular disease.

More than ten years ago, when I wrote *Fat or Fiction*, this was my primary message. It created a stir among dieticians and experts alike. I still hear arguments today, 'But you have to eat pasta!' In some ways

I think bread and pasta are more addictive than cigarettes. I really hope that as further studies reiterate the facts, the message will reach critical mass. *The biggest risk to our weight and our health is refined carbs and all fats are not evil!*

Low-fat diets are almost always high in carbs, so it's no coincidence that the fat phobia perpetuated in recent decades has fuelled our obesity epidemic. My advice? If you consume the appropriate amount of kilojoules (goal weight x 100) and get most of your carbs from vegetables, fruits and some wholegrains, the amount of fat in the diet doesn't matter nearly as much as you might think.

THE TRUTH **ABOUT FRUCTOSE**

In the forty years since the introduction into the food chain of high-fructose corn syrup as a cost-effective sweetener in the US, rates of obesity worldwide have skyrocketed. High-fructose corn syrup is found in a wide range of foods and beverages, including some fruit juices, soft drinks, cereal, bread, yoghurt, ketchup, salad dressings, confectionery, mayonnaise and even cough syrup. The US has one of the fattest populations in the world and Americans currently consume, on average, 27 kilos of the stuff per person every year! This number appears to be even higher in teenagers, who likely consume more soft drinks and juices.

If fructose is from fruit, it must be the preferred sweetener, right? Wrong! In fact, fructose is one of the worst sweeteners you can possibly consume. Table sugar (sucrose) is a combination of fructose and glucose. Studies that compare the effects of glucose and fructose consistently show that it is the fructose part of sugar that does the most damage, raising triglycerides (blood fats) and causing insulin resistance.

While some experts claim that fructose is no different from — or even preferable to — other sweeteners, a Princeton University research team recently demonstrated that all sweeteners are far from equal when it comes to weight gain. The study (Bartley G Hoebel, 'High-fructose corn syrup causes characteristic of obesity in rats: Increased body weight, body fat and triglyceride levels', Pharmacology Biochemistry and Behavior, 2010, DOI: 10.1016/j.pbb.2010.02.012) revealed that rats consuming high-fructose corn syrup gained significantly more weight than those that consumed table sugar, even with an identical calorie intake. In addition, long-term consumption of high-fructose corn syrup led to abnormal increases in body fat, particularly around the abdomen, and a rise in triglycerides.

'Some people have claimed that high-fructose corn syrup is no different than other sweeteners when it comes to weight gain and obesity, but our results make it clear that this just isn't true, at least under the conditions of our tests,' said the study's author, Princeton University psychology professor Bart Hoebel, who specialises in the neuroscience of appetite, weight and sugar addiction. 'When rats are drinking high-fructose corn syrup at levels well below those in soda pop, they're becoming obese — every single one, across the board. Even when rats are fed a high-fat diet, you don't see this; they don't all gain extra weight.'

The study monitored weight gain, body fat and triglyceride levels. Over a six-month period, the study compared rats eating their regular diet with rats on a diet rich in high-fructose corn syrup. The results revealed signs of a dangerous condition known as metabolic syndrome (also known as insulin resistance or syndrome X), a combination of medical disorders associated with insulin resistance including abnormal weight gain, a significant increase in blood fats and increased fat deposition, especially visceral fat (surrounding internal organs) around the belly. Those rats fed on high-fructose corn syrup gained 48 per cent more weight than those eating a normal diet.

Another study examined the effects of a high-fructose diet on the children of diabetics and non-diabetics, revealing that fructose increased triglycerides by a whopping 50 per cent in the children of non-diabetic patients as well. Deposits of fat in the liver increased in all groups by more than 75 per cent.

So how did fructose become so bad for us? Well, it began when we started messing about with nature. Fructose really belongs in fruit, where it's accompanied by fibre, vitamins and other natural goodies. Removed from its source and processed into a concentrated additive, it becomes metabolic poison.

The presence of fructose in some products will come as a surprise. I've noticed among new clients over the past few years that fructose intolerance appears to be increasing dramatically. To this end, I highly recommend that you read labels diligently and avoid the cheap fructose syrups and additives (derived from corn) at all costs.

TIPS TO **CUT BACK ON SUGAR**

» Take responsibility for your food choices and start reading labels. Don't be seduced by the marketing hype on the face of a product. Read the fine print. Better still, purchase food without any fine print, such as fresh fruit and vegetables.

» Check out the nutritional panel on a product before you purchase it. Find the grams of sugar and divide them by four. This will tell you how many teaspoons of sugar the product contains.

» Don't be seduced by sugars masquerading as 'healthy alternatives', such as raw sugar, organic sugar, brown sugar or even Manuka honey (all honey is very high in fructose). All of these will upset your blood sugar and are detrimental to health and your weight-loss efforts.

» Wean yourself off added sugars in tea, coffee or cereal. You'll find that when you go without for a while, you'll lose the taste for it. And it will make a huge difference to your waistline!

» Don't be gullible when it comes to low-fat or fat-free 'healthy' snacks. I can almost guarantee they'll be chock-full of sugar, not to mention a heap of 'empty' calories. Real unprocessed food is always best.

» The more colourful food you choose, the less 'white stuff' you'll be eating. The white stuff includes refined flours, sugars and processed grains. They're all identified as sugars in the body and, when consumed in excess (which is easily done), will make you fat.

» Be conscious that some artificial sweeteners can still cause cravings for sugar and carbs. They can also deplete your body of chromium, a necessary mineral for controlling blood sugar.

» Ditch the juice. It's just too much sugar in one hit.

» Limit fruit consumption to two pieces a day and try to avoid those higher in sugar, such as mangoes and grapes.

THE **GREAT PRETENDERS**

With all the hype surrounding weight loss and diets these days, it's not surprising to see a vast array of 'health food' options appearing on the shelves. Once reserved for speciality health-food stores, these products now have a strong presence in mainstream supermarkets. While more and more food manufacturers are jumping on the health-food bandwagon, how many of these foods are as virtuous as they claim to be and how many are simply masquerading as 'healthy'?

CEREAL

One of the most common health-food imposters is found in the cereal aisle. For years, breakfast cereals have been touted as the staple requirement for a healthy body. Sports people have been recruited to sing their praises. Some are even claimed to be 'ironman food'.

Sold as the best source of dietary fibre, most cereals are loaded with sugar and highly processed grains. Some are 'fortified' with all sorts of nutrients so we then assume they're even healthier.

Wholegrain cereals are better than many of the commercial varieties, but those who are sensitive to blood-sugar fluctuations will still need to be wary. I challenge you to find a commercial cereal that doesn't have a list of ingredients as long as your arm and doesn't contain some form of processed grains and added sugars. They're made to be inexpensive for high profit margins and to taste yummy so we eat more of them! As a rule, stick to cereals with less than 3 grams of sugar and more than 3 grams of fibre per serving. You'll be surprised how few cereals fit the bill.

So which cereal is the best choice? Good old-fashioned rolled oats. The list of ingredients will read 'oats', period. Rolled oats have less than 0.5 grams of sugar and 3.9 grams of fibre per serving. They can be made into porridge or mixed with nuts and seeds to create your own homemade muesli — yummy and healthy!

MUESLI BARS

Muesli bars are glorified confectionery. These 'great pretenders' are generally glued together with loads of sugar and highly processed carbs, with some overprocessed fats thrown in for good measure.

Don't be fooled by their 'health food' exterior. I am yet to find a muesli bar worthy of this title.

FRESH FISH

Salmon is an amazing source of omega-3 fats, which are essential for heart health, act as a natural anti-inflammatory and are involved in brain function, to name just a few of their many health benefits. Wild, deep-sea 'oily' fish are one of the best natural sources of omega-3.

When fish is farmed, away from its natural environment, it can contain a higher level of carcinogenic (cancer causing) chemicals such as polychlorinated biphenyls (PCBs). These chemicals can be used by farmers to kill off algae and are consequently absorbed into the flesh of the fish. PCBs build up in the human body and may cause serious health problems. Pregnant women and young children are most at risk, and PCBs can affect the development of an unborn baby's brain.

Antibiotics are also often used in the fish-farming process, potentially making us resistant to antibiotics and increasing our susceptibility to infection.

Mercury contamination is a widespread problem with certain fish. Large predatory fish at the top of the food chain, such as shark (flake) and swordfish, generally contain higher levels as their diet of smaller fish concentrates contamination.

So what about organic fish? Some organic fish farms are now starting to emerge. Wild fish cannot be certified as organic, as the full history of the fish cannot be known and their environment may be contaminated with pollutants.

At this stage I suggest you ask questions when purchasing fresh fish and go 'wild' or 'organic' where possible.

YOGHURT

'Real' yoghurt has many health benefits. It's high in calcium and live culture to help regulate our intestinal flora and support digestive health. Unfortunately, our taste buds become accustomed to sweetness over time so some people don't like the tart taste of natural yoghurt. Manufacturers began to add all sorts of flavours, colours, sugars and artificial sweeteners to our beloved yoghurt. We even have it in a probiotic sweet liquid form if we prefer.

The ironic thing about adding sugar to yoghurt is that sugar is the very thing that upsets our intestinal flora. 'Bad' bacteria thrive on sugar, yet we're adding it to our probiotics (the natural properties of yoghurt which encourage 'good' bacteria) for taste!

The low-fat revolution has meant more additives to our yoghurt. You've noticed the gelatinous texture of low-fat yoghurt compared with the thicker, creamier texture of the full-cream varieties? The taste and texture is generally plumped up with added thickeners and sweeteners. Personally, I prefer to have the real, natural product. Yep, full cream! Just have a smidge less.

The bottom line: if you're going to eat flavoured yoghurt you may as well eat ice-cream. Freeze it and it would be the same thing.

CANOLA (RAPESEED) OIL

Most of us have been led to believe that canola oil, and a variety of similar vegetable oils, are the healthy choice. But there are a few things you should know about our beloved oils. High temperatures are needed to extract canola oil from the rapeseed plant, turning any trace of omega-3 rancid. This foul-smelling rancidity now needs to be deodorised, often followed by caustic refining, degumming and bleaching. The heating process also has a high risk of producing dangerous trans fats.

Unless the label on an oil clearly states that it is 'cold pressed' and 'organic', leave it on the shelf.

MARGARINE

It's touted as being the healthy alternative to butter, but where does margarine come from? It's plant based, so it must be better for us, right? Margarine is possibly the greatest pretender of all, and it's recommended by doctors and the Heart Foundation to boot.

Margarine is a form of highly processed vegetable oil that's partially hydrogenated, a process that is used to make liquid oil semisolid at room temperature (so that it resembles butter) and is known to produce carcinogens. It's interesting to note that prior to the 1920s we ate plenty of lard, butter, beef and cheese — my mum used to spread lard on bread! — but both strokes and heart attacks were far less common than they are now. Since the introduction of hydrogenated oils, high omega-6 vegetable oils and tons of processed carbs, heart disease is now one of the most common causes of death in the Western world.

So should you choose margarine or butter? I must admit I don't consume either, but if I had to choose I'd definitely go for the less-processed alternative of butter.

JUICE

Fruit is great for you. Fruit juice, not so much. It would likely take around ten to twelve oranges to make a glass of freshly squeezed juice. It's unlikely you'd be able to eat ten to twelve oranges in one sitting, yet it's possible to consume the pure sugar from ten to twelve oranges, minus the natural pulp and fibre, and then eat breakfast! 'But it's natural sugar,' I hear you say. Natural or refined, sugar will still rot your teeth and make you fat. Eat the whole fruits or vegetables rather than drink the juice.

IN SUMMARY

To keep it simple: if you choose foods whose origin you can still recognise, you're on the right track. Ask yourself: does it grow that way? Choose foods as close to their natural form as possible — whole fruit and veggies rather than juice, wholegrain cereals, cold-pressed organic vegetable oils, natural unflavoured yoghurt and wild or organic fish … and avoid the 'great pretenders' like the plague.

DECEPTIVE 'HEALTH FOOD' LABELLING

When I first met Linda, my editor for *Fat or Fiction*, she was a little on the chubby side (unlike the svelte, fit girl she is today). She told me how she would wander around the supermarket doing her weekly grocery run munching a bag of banana lollies. 'They're 100 per cent fat free!' she exclaimed quite proudly. I recall the look of disbelief and disappointment on her face when I broke the news that they were full of sugar, which was certainly not going to help her to become 'fat free'.

People still boast about being on a fat-free diet, or being vegetarian, gluten free, sugar free or low carb, often with the primary purpose of losing weight or improving health. While some of us, such as diabetics and coeliacs, do have special dietary requirements, many of these foods are marketed more broadly as weight-loss alternatives and are displayed in the 'health food' aisle. It's important to note that while these foods may be suitable for individuals who need to restrict particular ingredients, this doesn't necessarily mean they are nutritionally superior, or 'healthy'.

The latest catchword? 'I've gone organic.' It instantly conjures up an image of green. Organic is equated with health and I agree that organic meat and vegetables are fine healthy options, but the market has gone well beyond those items now. There is organic ice-cream, muesli, honey, juice, bread and pasta. It's an organic world. This growing industry is worth millions annually, but we should be aware of what is hype and what is truth. Some manufacturers are quick to label their not-so-healthy food as organic.

Organic means 'produced without chemical fertilisers or pesticides', but this doesn't necessarily mean that organic foods are healthy. Organic foods can still contain sugar or trans fats. A multitude of artificial or processed ingredients may be added during the manufacture of organic processed foods, so 'organic' can only be considered one criterion for healthy food choices — not the only one.

A vegetarian or vegan diet precludes animal products but allows sugar, cakes, biscuits and highly starched processed food. Vegetarian snacks include sugar-laden sultanas, starchy lentil burgers and heavily processed two-minute noodles.

'Reduced fat' tends to mean less fat than the original product or its competitor, but these products can still be quite high in fat. It's all relative. The question you need to ask yourself is: 'less fat compared to what?' The resulting lack of taste and texture in lower fat products is often compensated for with sugars, thickeners and artificial ingredients. It's also important to note the type of fat in a product. If it's an unprocessed, 'healthy' form of fat, such as omega-3, lowering the fat grams would actually reduce the nutritional value.

Similarly, low-carb foods may just be lower in carbs than a competing brand or the 'regular' version of the product. They can be high in processed fats and artificial additives.

Sugar-free foods are rarely free of artificial sweeteners, which should be used sparingly. While the majority of artificial sweeteners won't upset your blood-sugar levels, many are chemical substances and not enough research has been done to look into possible long-term side effects to demonstrate that prolonged use doesn't cause harm over time. In particular, avoid using aspartame. Plant-derived stevia looks to be a preferred choice at this stage.

Gluten-free foods don't contain wheat or oats, so they are suitable for people with an allergy or intolerance to gluten. There's no guarantee the food in gluten-free products is healthy or made from unprocessed ingredients, and they're often plumped up with 'like' grain substitutes.

The marketing focus for all of these foods is what is not in them rather than what is. Always read the complete list of ingredients, not just the fat, calories or carbohydrates, and ask yourself whether organic ice-cream is a healthy food choice. (In case you're still wondering, the answer is no.)

PEER PRESSURE: **THE JUNK PUSHERS**

The week begins with a Sunday lunch celebrating your parents' anniversary — champagne, cake, rich sauces and warm bread rolls. 'Go on, it's a special occasion,' everyone says when you hesitate, reluctantly toasting with your champagne glass.

Monday is your colleague's birthday and everyone at work has put in for a Black Forest cake. 'Go on, just a sliver!'

Tuesday is film night with your friend, who wants to share a jumbo popcorn. 'Go on, it's only once a week.'

Wednesday is dinner at your local Thai for friends who are moving overseas. 'Go on, just this once won't hurt you.'

Thursday is a meeting at work with important new clients, complete with cupcakes, lemon tarts and milky coffee. 'Go on, everyone else is digging in.'

Friday is drinks after work to celebrate your favourite workmate's last day. 'Go on, your diet can start on Monday.'

And Saturday? Well, Saturday is always a special occasion.

As regular as our social lives may be there is still a bizarre need to make every engagement an event. Of course, some occasions are special but they don't need junk food to prove it. If you start to cave in to these justifications, you may as well spatula a cream cake directly on to your belly and bypass your digestive tract.

Your friends and family shouldn't turn into junk pushers at these occasions if they want to support your choices. They often want you to drink, eat cakes and popcorn as a way of sharing the experience, and may appear dejected if you decline the offer, as though you are somehow rejecting them.

Junk pushers can be one of the most sensitive issues for people trying to lose weight and maintain a healthy lifestyle. We don't want to offend them, we care about them and want to take part in the celebration — we just don't want to eat cake. After making it through the tough launching weeks when you're just feeling as though you have kicked the sugar habit, the thought of a 'pre-change' food can make you feel nauseous. Eating it probably will make you feel nauseous, with an instant 'food hangover' headache to add to your woes.

Insulin levels have started to stabilise by this time, clothes are feeling looser and triumph is in the air. Then, the cake comes out and the peer pressure snowballs. The person offering you the food often can't keep your knock-back to herself, announcing to everyone that you're on a diet. All eyes turn to your waistline as some guests guiltily put down their creamy cakes and others claim the one we all love: 'You don't need to lose weight — go on, it's a special occasion.' You blush, and can either buckle under the weight of glaring eyes or stay resolute.

Generally we are the best judge of whether we need to lose a few excess kilos or improve our health — our body, our decision. And there will always be a special occasion. If you allow that to determine your food choices, you will never reach your goals.

Go to the parties, enjoy whatever food you feel able to eat or, better still, eat before you go so nothing will tempt you, but don't compromise your hard work and discipline for others. They may be caring, wanting you to share in the fun, and, unfortunately, they may also want to obstruct your resolve.

Keep alcohol consumption to moderate levels and remember that red wine is the best choice. Ask yourself if the cake will be good enough to wear on your belly for the next few months, or whether you'd rather fit into a new pair of jeans and be running around with lean abs. I think you'd agree that would be one hell of a special occasion.

HYPOTHETICAL #1

THE PROBLEM

Emma has been steadily gaining weight each year since having her two children. Between caring for her sons and holding down a part-time job, she has little time to devote to a structured gym program. She is also concerned she needs more energy than she could muster on a restrictive and regimented diet plan.

THE SOLUTION

DIET

Getting organised is key. It's important to set some rules around the house, such as the following:

» Don't eat standing up! It sounds pretty obvious, but Emma really does need to 'sit and chew'. If she's going to have a snack, she needs to put it on a plate and sit at the table. It's all the unconscious 'inhalation' of ingredients while preparing meals for the family which add the kilos. Emma can keep some washed and peeled veggie sticks in a container in the fridge for snacking on.

» Instead of sipping on a glass of Chardonnay while preparing dinner, switch to a wine glass with sparkling mineral water and a fresh lime wedge.

» Emma needs to think about where she'll be and what she'll be doing tomorrow and ensure she has healthy options readily available. Cook a little extra dinner and save it for tomorrow's lunch.

» Even if Emma is choosing healthy foods, it will be impossible to shed the kilos if she's eating twice as much as she needs. Portions are important, so make use of kitchen scales to keep serving sizes in check. She will quickly develop an 'eye' for appropriate portions.

» Some of the most common 'hidden' extras to watch out for are milky coffee (even skinny, without sugar), juices, 'healthy' salads laden with dressing, low-fat yoghurt (filled with sugar) and consuming too many nuts.

» Curb takeaways to only once a week at most, and try to opt for the lesser of evils, such as grilled fish and salad rather than battered, fried fish and chips. If pizza is on the menu, avoid thick, cheesy bases— better still, avoid bases entirely and go for the topping. A rotisserie chicken is a great takeaway choice along with a delicious Greek salad. There are ways to find a happy medium when it comes to takeaways, which will minimise the risk of undoing all of that good work.

» Invest in a water jug (preferably a filter jug) and use this to gauge how much water is consumed over the course of the day. Whether at home or at work, aim to empty a 2-litre jug each and every day. If this proves difficult, aim for a litre before lunch and polish off the second litre by dinnertime. Sometimes a wedge of fresh lime or even a splash of diet cordial can help.

STRENGTH

Three thirty-minute sessions a week. That's all it takes!

» As Emma has very little time, she would likely find a trip to the gym a bit of a chore. It's important to make any exercise convenient and time efficient, so three times a week Emma has the choice of either following an exercise DVD at home while the boys have a nap, or taking the kids to the park and playing with them on the playground equipment. I know it sounds a little silly, but what fun! There are many strength exercises that can be performed at home without the need for any equipment at all, such as squats (twenty repetitions of sitting on a chair will get those legs burning), sit-ups on the floor, holding a 'plank' or 'bridge' position to develop core strength, and basic push-ups. If three thirty-minute sessions a week are not feasible, fifteen minutes every day is also a very effective option.

CARDIO

Thirty minutes a day, every day

» Emma's not keen on running (and neither is her pelvic floor), so walking is ideal — particularly when she can push a pram for a little extra resistance. It doesn't matter if she has one thirty-minute walk, two fifteen-minute walks or three ten-minute walks per day. The message is: just move. Every bit of walking she can fit in is worthwhile. If getting outdoors proves to be a struggle, she could hire a treadmill or a stationary bike at home for a 'plan B'.

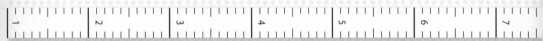

TEN FIT-BODY SECRETS

I think I've heard every excuse under the sun as to why we can't lose weight. Women invariably think they're eating too much fat and men think they're not exercising enough. No-one ever thinks they have time. Sometimes they're right but the extent of misinformation continues to be staggering.

Weight loss essentially takes simple common sense, though there are some ways to make it easier to adhere to your commitments and save your ever-precious time. These are my Golden Fat Loss Rules and they are based on experience, research and years of feedback from readers and clients.

1. **REGULATE PORTION SIZES** Check the menu section of this book to find your category type and follow the appropriate portion amounts. 'All you can eat' is never an option, even if it's healthy food.

2. **EXERCISE CONSISTENTLY** Walking for thirty minutes can easily be worked into the busiest days. Strength training is essential for maintaining muscle and therefore boosting metabolism.

3. **SET REALISTIC GOALS** Don't aim too high, just aim fairly. If you want too much too soon, you'll be disappointed and deterred. It's far better to expect less while being realistic: you'll be pleasantly surprised with every small, valuable gain you make.

4. **THINK BODY COMPOSITION** Think less about how much you weigh on the scales and more about the fat–lean weight ratio. Being 'light' does not necessarily mean you are lean or heading in the right direction. Remember, extreme diet and exercise regimes are likely to make you *lighter* yet *fatter*.

5. **VALUE PROTEIN** Protein really is the building block of life. It's also a great way to curb your appetite and cravings, as well as stabilise your blood-sugar levels. Protein feeds muscle so that it's not only retained but also improves in conditioning, helping to create your new shape. 'High' protein is not necessary (or healthy). Adequate amounts of protein in each of our main meals is the ideal balance.

6. **AVOID SUGAR AND REFINED 'WHITE' FOODS** Refined foods are void of nutrition but incredibly high in calories, offering very little value but plenty of padding for your waistline. Processing grains and plant foods creates a product dense in calories yet low in fibre, which means we can consume more and still not feel full.

7. **RELY LESS ON MOTIVATION AND MORE ON INSPIRATION** Generally, motivation is a temporary, superficial urge. It can start as an external impetus — a special function, a beach holiday or a yearning to fit into your favourite pair of jeans — but eventually it's down to you, your discipline, your priorities and your belief in yourself. Contrary to popular belief, this is very different from inspiration. To be inspired generally has a much deeper, more meaningful, compelling and long-term foundation. Maybe it's to be a role model for your children, or to achieve a personal physical challenge. Ask yourself how your life would change for the better if you were brimming with health, energy and confidence. Dig deep, find what inspires you and write it down.

8. **TAKE RESPONSIBILITY** There is nothing to be gained in deluding yourself and pretending you have been sticking to healthy guidelines when you've been munching on nuggets every other day, or kidding yourself that those teeny-weeny bits of biscuit that you break off every time you go past the pantry don't really add up to anything. If you continue to blame someone or something else, then that logic will have you believing that it will be up to someone or something else to solve the problem. And we both know that will never happen. Remember, what you eat in private shows up in public.

9. **EXERCISE** Activity has to become part of your life, not a chore that you dread or begrudge. Always begin with exercise you enjoy and you will stick to it, with pleasure and great results. If you can't find something you enjoy, do it anyway. I'm sure you don't love brushing your teeth or showering, but you wouldn't dream of not performing these daily rituals. For some reason, when it comes to exercise we give ourselves the option to 'feel like it' or not. I have never heard anyone tell me they've regretted going for a walk or dragging their lazy butt to the gym. You know that no matter how much you 'don't feel like it', you will always feel better once you've made the effort.

10. **REJECT FADS** There really is no magic bullet but there are as many new fads bursting on to the market as there are overweight people to succumb to them. You are not out of shape due to a fad-diet deficiency, so don't anticipate that the 'missing link' will come along and turn you into Angelina or Brad.

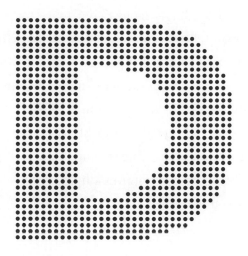

BALANCE THROUGH THE AGES

Despite passing the big four-O mark a few years back, I feel quite comfortable with my age. I can now quote that old adage, 'If only I knew then what I know now.' I feel stronger and fitter than I was in my twenties. So far, I haven't booked in for cougar pole-dancing lessons or lip collagen, so I guess I didn't experience the dreaded 'crisis' I'd been so fiercely warned about (perhaps it's still to come!).

One thing I have noticed, however, is the gradual but definite changes in the way my body reacts to food and exercise. What used to keep me in shape doesn't quite cut it these days. I need to be a bit more diligent with consistency when it comes to exercise. I'm not necessarily referring to weight gain on the scales, but rather changes to my body composition. I've learned the hard way that my body becomes 'soft' at a startlingly rapid rate if I take my eye off the ball. I've also heard many clients comment about this type of shift in their own bodies. Changes tend to happen throughout various phases of our lives, but they have become increasingly obvious to me since I entered my fifth decade. So the question is, what do we need to do to curb this process and how does our lifestyle need to adjust for us to navigate our way through while staying in good shape? Well, I can tell you I'm not going down without a fight.

The younger you start, the better.

TODDLERS **TO TWEENS**

These are the crucial years to help establish a healthy future. Our body is in overdrive when it comes to growth and development and our fat cells are at their most responsive, readily multiplying if stimulated by overeating. This can potentially perpetuate a weight battle, now and well into adult life. Overfat children will generally be overfat adults, so cut the 'puppy fat' justification.

EAT

Kids at this age are often 'too busy' to sit down and eat a meal. They are easily seduced by marketing campaigns and peer pressure and are often reluctant to eat their veggies. The question you need to ask is: are your kids getting enough vital nutrients? It may be time to get creative with food presentation. Involve the kids in shopping for fresh produce and preparing it. Do whatever it takes.

Calcium is best known for optimising bone growth and contributing to a fracture-free skeleton throughout all life stages. Most of us are aware that calcium is found in bones, but it also circulates in the bloodstream, playing a vital role in normal heart rhythm, blood clotting and muscle function.

It's common for children, especially teens, to be calcium deficient. Soft drinks and juices have infiltrated kids' diets, causing milk intake to decrease. The high phosphate levels in carbonated drinks lower calcium levels in the blood. Caffeine, which is found in some soft drinks, acts as a diuretic, causing excessive calcium excretion via the urine. Added to this, calcium needs increase dramatically at a time in life when kids, especially girls, get far less than the suggested amount. One study found that adolescent girls averaged only 60 per cent of their daily requirement. Just before the teen years, and all throughout adolescence, children must get enough calcium to provide the foundation for strong bones as this is the time our bodies form almost half of the bone mass we will ever have.

Our kids need three servings of dairy each day. One serving is equivalent to 250 mL of milk, 200 grams of yoghurt or 40 grams of cheese.

On-the-go lifestyles are one of the reasons why kids are eating less fibre than they should. This is primarily due to a higher consumption of processed fast foods and fewer home-cooked meals, which can lead to changes in our taste buds and a consequent aversion to fresh fruit and vegetables. Fibre is necessary for stimulating the gut to pass waste with greater ease. Fibre also helps us feel fuller. Generally speaking, high-fibre plant foods are rich in vitamins and minerals to fuel growth and development. They also contain beneficial plant compounds called phytonutrients, which boost your child's immunity. To calculate your child's daily fibre needs in grams, add five to his or her age. For example, a ten-year-old requires 15 grams of daily dietary fibre.

Magnesium is involved in about 300 bodily functions responsible for keeping your child healthy. This essential mineral helps maintain normal muscle, nerve and heart function, and improves our immune system, energy production and bone health. Offering your kids dark-green vegetables, a variety of nuts and seeds and wholegrains will help them meet their magnesium needs.

As a powerful antioxidant nutrient, vitamin E battles free radicals and exposure to ultraviolet rays, air pollution and cigarette smoke. Vitamin E is also vital for a strong immune system. Vitamin E is found in abundance in fatty foods, so reducing fat intake for fear of weight gain can hinder healthy eating in kids, as can restricting nuts. Unrefined vegetable oils, walnuts and dark-green leafy vegetables are rich in vitamin E.

Potassium ensures normal heart and muscle function, maintains fluid balance, contributes to energy production and promotes strong bones. Just like adults, kids generally don't eat enough fresh plant foods. Dairy foods, fresh lean meats and seafood are also good sources of potassium. As a general rule, the more processed the food, the more sodium and less potassium it contains.

If your child is battling a weight issue, reduce sugars and processed carbs. Focus on healthy wholefoods, eliminate snacking on sugar-laden 'treats' between meals and increase daily activity and sports.

MOVE

Daily — any and all activities are great for a healthy mind and body. Activities need to be fun (as they do at any age).

SLEEP

Primary school children need about nine to ten hours of sleep a night. Studies show that increasing your child's sleep by as little as half an hour can dramatically improve school performance.

RULES

- » Have regular meals.

- » Eat fish for optimum brain function.

- » Focus on nutrient-rich, colourful meals.

- » Cut back on the processed 'white' foods.

- » Eliminate soft drinks and sugary juices.

- » Increase water intake.

- » Sleep for nine to ten hours a night.

- » Don't leave the house without breakfast.

MID-TO-LATE TEENS

With hormones raging, peer pressure increasing and study becoming more intense, teenagers face a high-risk period for their health, fitness and body composition to dramatically decline. Combine this with all-too-common highly processed fast foods and we have a recipe for disaster.

EAT

At this stage, peer pressure is rife and unfortunately some healthy foods can be very 'uncool'. A healthy diet is not something that most teenagers give much thought to. Teenage years are commonly a time when meals are skipped, more food is eaten away from home and less-nutritious snacks are eaten, often in excess. It's common for teens to lack the skills and motivation to do what they should to stay healthy. Skipping meals, especially breakfast, and choosing processed and convenience foods over fresh translates into too much processed fat, sodium and sugar, and not enough of the fibre, vitamins and minerals essential to their health now and later. Calcium needs are higher than ever during the teen years — 1300 milligrams a day. Teens require the calcium equivalent of three to four servings of dairy each day.

Hydration is crucial for optimum physical and mental alertness during intense study periods. Even a small degree of dehydration can cause lethargy, mental 'fogginess' and cravings for caffeine or sweet snacks in the struggle to boost energy.

Iron, as a component of red blood cells, is necessary for carrying oxygen to every cell in the body. Iron deficiency is common in adolescent girls and people who limit meat. Menstruating young women are at increased risk of an iron shortfall because their diets may not contain enough iron-rich foods to make up for monthly losses. Adolescents often feel pressure to limit what they eat so that they can conform to a certain look. They may also restrict food intake to achieve a certain weight for a sport or for social events.

You want your fourteen-year-old to lay off the fries and learn to love broccoli. Why? Because you know that eating vegetables is linked to a lower risk of developing chronic conditions such as cancer and heart disease later in life. That may motivate you to pile your plate with greens, but it probably won't sway your 'invincible' teen. Avoid power struggles over food. Strict control over what a child eats can backfire. Teens may respond by over- or under-eating just to assert independence.

SLEEP

Sleep is as important to all of us as food and water, but most of us don't get enough of it. It's no surprise that insufficient or poor-quality sleep causes varying degrees of fatigue. When fatigued, we become accident-prone, our judgement is impaired and we're more likely to make mistakes and irrational decisions. Staying awake for twenty-four hours leads to disorientation similar to that of a drunken state. So it's fair to say that lack of sleep can affect a teenager's school performance and could also be linked to behavioural and emotional problems, such as depression. Lack of sleep reduces your attention span, slows normal reaction time, impairs memory and judgement, reduces motivation and increases the likelihood of moodiness. Sleepy kids tend to 'speed up' rather than slow down, displaying moodiness and emotional overreaction at the slightest provocation.

Obviously there are many causes of sleep deprivation, ranging from personal priorities to stress, sleep disorders, diet, medication or environmental factors such as noise and light. In the case of teenagers, the culprit is commonly a combination of an ever-busy social life (sitting up half the night on Facebook), stress and poor time management.

Chronically sleep-deprived teenagers are more likely to have problems with impulse control, which leads to risk-taking behaviours. Lack of sleep is also strongly associated with increased risk of disorders such as depression and attention deficit hyperactivity disorder (ADHD). Studies show that high-school students who regularly score low in school tests and assignments get, on average, half an hour less sleep per night than high-school students who regularly get high marks.

Teenagers need about nine to ten hours' sleep. There is evidence that around puberty there is a shift in the sleep–wake cycle to being sleepy later in the evening with a preference for waking later in the morning. To improve sleep, avoid caffeinated beverages, improve the sleeping environment — the room should be dark and soundproof — and remove distractions such as computers, mobiles and TVs from the bedroom (good luck with that one!).

MOVE

As study becomes more intense, stress levels increase and teens become increasingly sedentary. Many teens are involved in sports, but plenty still don't get the minimum thirty to sixty minutes of recommended daily activity. Physical activity improves endurance and muscle strength, builds strong bones and joints, and promotes wellbeing. Moving around also helps maintain a healthy weight. Many research studies have concluded that a lack of vigorous exercise is a primary cause for obesity in children. There is a very good chance that an overweight teenager will become an overweight adult.

RULES

» Drink plenty of water (your weight divided by 28 will give you your required daily amount in litres).

» Sleep for nine to ten hours a night.

» Don't skip breakfast.

» Ensure adequate consumption of essential fats for healthy skin, general health and brain function.

» Ensure adequate intake of iron, magnesium, zinc and B-complex vitamins to counteract stress and facilitate growth — in other words, lean protein, colourful plant foods and wholegrains.

TURBULENT TWENTIES

This is the decade of change, when we've left school and, often, home. Mum's no longer doing our cooking. We're working longer hours and still adjusting to all of this change. Time management and organisation are of the essence.

EAT

If you haven't already, it's time to learn how to cook! In my experience, if you become proficient at cooking you won't find 'healthy' food boring or monotonous. If necessary, take a few cooking lessons, learn about new ingredients and experiment. You may surprise yourself. Like anything, once you become proficient, food preparation becomes quicker, easier and more enjoyable.

It's common for twenty-somethings to be burning the candle at both ends. You're likely enjoying the peak of your social life and simultaneously getting stuck into your career. The need for good nutrition is as important now as ever. Similar to a teenager's requirements, focus on lean protein, colourful fresh plant foods and essential fats. However, now that your body has finished growing and your work may make you more sedentary, it's time to pay particular attention to portion control (check the menu guide for appropriate amounts). The bottom line? Keep it simple. Eat real ingredients and don't be seduced by fads.

ALCOHOL

Yes, in your twenties I've added a category dedicated specifically to alcohol. We all know that overconsumption is detrimental to our health and our weight, but we're invincible in our twenties, right?

From an energy perspective, one standard (100 mL) glass of wine provides 80 to 100 calories. For those of you with an appreciation of 'fishbowl' wineglasses, there are supposed to be around six glasses in a bottle, not two! Translated into exercise, it will take you twenty minutes of brisk walking to burn off a single standard glass. Even if you do try to counteract overconsumption with more walking, why exercise just to break even? You may as well reduce the alcohol and actually burn some fat for your efforts. Put simply, more than five standard drinks over a week is likely to result in excess fat storage — particularly around your belly. And before you ask, no, you can't have them all in one night and, no, you can't save them up and have them all in three weeks' time!

MOVE

Chances are your working day is now longer and more sedentary than when you were in your teens. Rather than meeting friends after work for drinks or coffee, try a 'walk and talk'. That's right, instead of sitting and consuming yet more calories, burn them off as you chat. Try walking to and from work, or at least parking a little further away. It all adds up. Take up tennis lessons with a friend, walk the dog or join a class at your local gym — whatever it takes to keep you motivated and in routine.

Now that your body has finished growing, it will start to age more rapidly if you make poor choices. In our twenties we tend to take better care of our material possessions than our body. Remember, you only get one, so take good care of it. Contrary to popular belief, you're not invincible.

SLEEP

As adults, we need about eight hours' sleep, depending on individual factors. We tend to need less sleep as we get older, but be guided by your own state of alertness. At the risk of sounding like my mother, if you feel tired during the day, aim to get more sleep. You'll find that you function better on every level, plus you'll have more energy to exercise.

RULES

» Time to be a grown-up. Work on developing your new independent routine: time management, exercise, food preparation and cooking.

» Don't cut out any of the major food groups in an attempt to lose weight.

» Avoid fad diets like the plague. They're targeting you!

» Get at least eight hours' sleep a night and make up for 'sleep debt' whenever necessary.

» Move for at least thirty to sixty minutes each day.

THIRTY-SOMETHING

Not only are you likely to be in the midst of your career, you may also have children of your own, or they're now a consideration. As your life and your body start to change, so too will your food and exercise needs. For women, it is said that perimenopause can begin as early as thirty-five, so it's common in this decade for our body to start reacting a little differently. We also lose around 3 per cent of lean muscle each decade from the age of twenty-five if we don't use it. This, combined with the consequent lowering of your metabolic rate (due to muscle loss), a busy lifestyle, hormonal changes and, for women, possible pregnancies, puts you at high risk of becoming overfat.

EAT

Your body may have started responding a little differently than it did in your twenties. Due to extended work and family commitments, you may be a little more sedentary and you may have lost a bit of lean muscle tissue, which has allowed your metabolic rate to drop (not to mention your backside). It's time to reel in the routine and put some focus back on your body maintenance. This means investing in a set of kitchen scales and monitoring your food portion sizes. Even if you're choosing all the right foods, if you're consuming twice as much as you need, you will still be gaining weight or preventing fat loss. Increase the amount of colourful fresh plant food you consume. Raw, cooked — a variety of both is best.

Women who are planning on a family should consider supplementing their diet with folic acid, as well as essential fats (from fish, as well as flaxseed oil). During pregnancy, the foetus requires omega-3 fats to develop a normal brain. Once breastfeeding begins, mum has no omega-3 left for her own brain function. There are now several studies showing a link between an omega-3 deficiency and postnatal depression. Use (refrigerated) flaxseed oil on salads and wherever you're using oil uncooked, and consume fresh fish such as salmon, sardines and tuna at least twice a week and you should be covered. Keep in mind that large fish, such as swordfish and shark, can be contaminated with high levels of toxic metals, such as PCBs, dioxins and mercury, so excessive consumption is not recommended. It's also advisable to check the label on fish oil supplements. If the manufacturer has gone to the trouble of testing for and removing contaminants, they will certainly tell you all about it on the packaging.

MOVE

A consistent routine of weight-bearing exercise is now absolutely essential. You will no longer 'get away with' spasmodic bouts of being a gym junkie. It's now a case of use it or you will quite literally lose it (muscle, that is). To keep your metabolism firing on all cylinders, you must participate in some form of strength training two to three times a week. This is anything that makes your muscles work, such as weight training, bodyweight exercises, boxing, circuit classes … whatever floats your boat. And no, you won't become a muscle-bound hulk. It takes big weights to build big muscles, and as a novice you won't be able to lift weights that heavy, let alone train with them. It takes at least three to five years of dedication to consistent heavy weight training for someone, male or female, to gain significant muscle size — and even then, you will most likely be limited by your genetic potential.

RULES

» Walk (or undertake equivalent low- to moderate-intensity cardio activity) *every day* for thirty to forty-five minutes. Yep, seven days!

» Do strength training two to three times a week.

» Be conscious of portion sizes (see the menu guide for accurate individual requirements).

» Reduce alcohol consumption to a maximum of five standard drinks a week — and not all in one day.

» Consume lean protein with each of your three main meals for satiety and retention of lean muscle.

» Don't be seduced by fads.

FIT AT **FORTY**

Well, this one is now pretty close to home for me, although I still feel like I'm twenty-five. During our forties we may have let exercise slide in favour of career success or family commitments. Most women's bodies are moving towards some pretty dramatic hormone changes in this decade. Before you know it, you could be 'fat and forty' — never a good combination.

In my experience it's also a time when we start to take stock of what's important to us and, inevitably, a healthy body is high on the list. You've probably figured out by now that you're not invincible. If you haven't, it's time. You're now more likely to be seeing changes in your fat distribution. At this age it tends to concentrate mainly around the waist, which from a health perspective is the most dangerous place to store fat. The factors that influence this are hormonal changes, overconsumption (of alcohol and food) and stress.

EAT

It's likely that you're less active than you were in your twenties or thirties (which, of course, is not ideal or recommended). Your metabolic rate has probably taken a dive along with your exercise regime. It's crucial that you start to pay more attention to your food choices, even when you're not in an ideal routine (due to work functions, for instance).

If you try to be perfect you will fail every time. You need to establish a healthier daily regime that you can continue for the long term. That's right — permanent lifestyle changes. For women, you're preparing your body for an event of Olympic proportions: menopause. The healthier and better nourished your body is, the better you'll cope with the changes. For men, it's time to rein in the boozy work lunches and the sausages and beer at weekend barbecues. While I don't expect you to eat mung beans and tofu burgers, it's time to consider a happy medium.

MOVE

This is the decade in which our risk of heart disease, cancer, obesity and diabetes escalates. It's not a matter of not having time to exercise — you actually don't have time not to. Make the decision to move for at least thirty minutes a day, seven days a week. Your joints may not be what they used to be, particularly if you played impact sport (or, heaven forbid, attended '80s aerobics classes) in your younger years, so choose lower-impact exercise: walking, boxing, weight training, bodyweight training, using elliptical trainers, perhaps even a game of tennis with friends. I haven't written off our vintage to the retirement village just yet, but you have to start being realistic about what your body is capable of. One thing is for certain: you'll never find time to exercise. You have to make time. And if you haven't had a health check for a while (cholesterol, blood pressure, etc.), it's time.

RULES

» Keep to a strong routine of three balanced meals a day, with two optional snacks between (if needed).

» Make time to exercise for at least thirty minutes a day, seven days a week.

» Focus on portion sizes and don't pick or overindulge.

» Do some form of strength training two to three times a week, religiously.

» Focus on the quality of foods consumed. Cut the 'white' stuff.

» Eat essential fats — they're essential. Your heart and joints need them daily.

FIFTY **AND BEYOND**

Health risk factors are now at their peak but they don't have to be our destiny. The more you care for your body, the more resilient it will be. In our fifties, women generally experience a significant change in fat distribution, shifting to more of an apple shape (fat stored around the waist). Male distribution of body fat is generally concentrated around the waist throughout life, but now is the time it's likely to be getting a little out of control.

It doesn't have to be this way. Excess fat will be stored around the waist if excess fat is stored, but it's ultimately dependent on your lifestyle and your food choices. Many clients tell me that although they weighed 60 kilos when they were twenty, now that they're older that weight is unrealistic. 'Perhaps now 70 kilos is more feasible, right?' Wrong! Both men and women should expect to weigh less as we get older, not more. Our bone density and muscle tissue diminish and so too should our weight. Excess fat is stored over time and, presto!, you weigh 10 kilos more. If you were 60 kilos in your twenties, you certainly shouldn't be aiming for any more than that now … unless you intend to gain 10 kilos or so of lean muscle.

EAT

Calcium, lean protein and essential fats have never been more important to good health than they are now. Eating fish and flaxseed oil regularly will help to keep your heart and joints healthy. Daily consumption of dairy products will keep your bones healthy, and lean protein will help preserve your lean muscle and consequently your metabolism.

It's very common these days to be deficient in vitamin D. This can occur at any age, but people in their fifties and beyond tend to be more conscious of sun damage so need to supplement. Vitamin D can to be found in foods such as dairy products, oily fish, cod-liver oil and eggs. A combination of heeding warnings about exposure to harmful UV rays, our often fat-phobic diets and, paradoxically, rising obesity rates has seen vitamin D levels fall precariously low. (In a recent study, the more participants weighed the lower their vitamin D levels tended to be, which may be because vitamin D is a fat-soluble vitamin— Lagunova Z et al., 'Serum 25-hydroxyvitamin D is a predictor of serum 1,25-dihydroxyvitamin D in overweight and obese patients', The Journal of Nutrition, January 2011, 141(1), pp. 112–17.) Symptoms of vitamin D deficiency may be subtle, but can materialise as general pain and weakness. Low blood levels of vitamin D have been associated with cardiovascular disease, cancer, cognitive impairment in older adults and severe asthma in children.

MOVE

The loss of muscle and bone density will now accelerate for both men and women as growth and sex hormones diminish. It is absolutely imperative to train your muscles consistently to lower your risk of losing valuable muscle (and metabolic rate) and bone density, to fight excess fat and to maintain good cardiovascular health. A daily thirty-minute walk is a great start, but you'll have to hit the gym (or at least find a weight-bearing activity) two to three times a week to get the full benefits.

Our joints are generally not 100 per cent once we're over fifty, so high-impact exercise, such as jogging, is generally not ideal unless you're a seasoned runner. Lower-impact cardiovascular exercise is ideal — walking is brilliant. You can still walk at a fast pace and over a more challenging terrain to increase intensity without affecting your joints.

We're generally a lot 'younger' at fifty these days than we were several decades ago, but it's still very common to have joint degeneration or back or knee issues. If you don't enjoy a particular exercise or it irritates an old injury, find an alternative. It may be worth your while hiring a reputable personal trainer to assist you to develop an appropriate exercise program.

SLEEP

We often get less sleep as we get older. That's because our ability to sleep for long periods of time and to achieve the deep, restful stages of sleep decreases with age. In this age bracket it's common for us to have more fragile sleep, as we are more easily disturbed by light, noise and pain than when we were younger.

RULES

- » Don't be fat phobic. Consume essential fats for heart, skin and brain health.

- » Do weight-bearing exercises two to three times a week.

- » Perform some form of low-impact cardiovascular exercise for thirty minutes a day, seven days a week.

- » Be conscious of meal portion sizes and consume lean protein with each of the three main meals.

- » Take a multivitamin and mineral supplement daily to ensure optimum nutritional absorption.

- » Aim for a solid eight hours' sleep a night.

ACHIEVING YUMMY MUMMY-NESS!

Pregnancy may bring immeasurable joy to most women but postnatal bodies introduce a sour note to those who feel like not-so-yummy mummies.

Pregnancy is often blamed for weight gain even ten years on. How many times have I heard pregnancy blamed for excess weight gain and it just grew from there. I wonder how it grew.

Let's face it: we have a lot to live up to these days. Posh, Gwyneth, Elle, fifty-something supermum Madonna and hundreds of other much less famous supermums I've met over the years don't have similar complaints. Okay, I hear you saying, 'But they have nannies, trainers, chefs, more time … of course they can snap back into shape!' I can't dispute the truth in this, but it does go to show that, with the right advice, you can be a confident yummy mummy!

It's true that some hormones can become a bit out of whack after a woman gives birth, and there is a justifiable weight gain and change in fat distribution during pregnancy, but many of us hide behind our bumps and use them as an excuse to eat everything under the sun. Even foods a woman would never have touched pre-pregnancy turn up on the menu and the common justification is that she is 'eating for two' — two fully grown adults?

Sticking with the roomy baby-doll maternity frock and stretchy pants may allow you to continue to munch on chocolate and cheekily ascribe all bad choices to cravings, but excessive weight gain doesn't have to be a part of bearing children. What's more, now that you know more about epigenetics and how your lifestyle habits can affect your unborn child, you have even more reasons not to blow out before, during or after pregnancy.

If you chose instead to wear more fitted maternity fashion, your beautiful bump can remain just that: a bump, albeit a bump that grows in size. Hips, thighs, shoulders or any other areas of the body should only gain in size minimally during pregnancy and certainly return to some degree of normality soon after birth.

Get the all-clear from your doctor and feel confident about exercising in some form or another for as long as you feel comfortable, which in many cases may be right up until delivery, especially if you've exercised regularly for some time before becoming pregnant.

For others, light walks and swimming may be all that can be managed as the delivery time nears. The crucial factor is to listen to your body clearly and keep exercising and eating clean, unprocessed foods. Everything you are putting in your mouth you're feeding to your baby, so highly processed foods are well and truly off the menu.

To be safe when exercising from the second trimester onwards, keep track of your heart rate and make sure it doesn't accelerate too high. In the second trimester the heart rate should not exceed 140 bpm and by the third trimester — when the focus is on getting maximum nutrition to the baby — the heart rate shouldn't go beyond 120 bpm. You must also be aware of your body temperature, not allowing it to creep up too high. Stay well hydrated and never exercise in the heat.

It's safe to continue with a progressively modified weight-training regime throughout pregnancy, but gradually lighten the weights or decrease the number of repetitions and lengthen the rest period between sets. I would highly recommend this is supervised, or at the very least designed by a reputable fitness professional.

It is crucial to maintain muscle strength at this time — think of all the lifting that will be a routine part of your life once the baby is born. Strength, fitness and endurance will also be helpful during the delivery. Be sure to have your back well supported when lifting weights and if possible work with a personal trainer to ensure proper technique is maintained. It is not the time to be coping with an injury or overexerting yourself.

It would not be advisable to start strenuous exercise after you become pregnant. Even if you have jogged regularly or been part of a volleyball, basketball, netball or tennis team before pregnancy, these sports should certainly be stopped by the end of the second trimester. Lighter exercise such as moderate walking for twenty to thirty minutes every day and gentle, modified strength training are more advisable.

In summary, here are some of the advantages of staying fit during and post-pregnancy.

» Exercise decreases the risk of excess body fat postpartum.

» An emphasis on health and fitness during pregnancy will improve the physical and mental wellbeing of you and your baby.

» Maintaining a strong body will reduce the incidence of back pain and may provide for an easier labour.

» A focus on good nutrition will not only keep your body in shape and allow you to bounce back to pre-pregnancy size sooner, it will also provide your baby with the best tools for developing a healthy mind and body at this crucial stage of growth and development.

» Exercise will stimulate and improve circulation and reduce the incidence of fluid retention and related problems.

WHAT EXERCISES SHOULD I AVOID DURING PREGANCY?

» Avoid exercise that incorporates bending from the waist (may cause dizziness, heartburn and discomfort).

» Abandon overhead lifting exercises (your lower back is vulnerable to injury).

» Abandon exercise in the supine position (on your back) after the first trimester — this position may obstruct venous blood flow and cause dizziness, as well as reduced blood flow to the baby.

» Avoid erratic or excessively intense workouts — slow your workout pace to accommodate your increased heart rate and avoid overheating.

Don't let pregnancy be an excuse to overeat and stop moving. It will be a much more comfortable and enjoyable process if you eat well and move carefully and moderately so that you are well prepared for the high-intensity work of being a mum.

If you are considering starting a family, I would highly recommend getting yourself fit and strong beforehand to ensure a healthy pregnancy and postpartum recovery. You'll be giving your baby the best shot at a lifetime of good health. I think you'll agree that this reward is priceless.

SLEEP YOURSELF SLIM

Many of us underestimate the importance of sleep: what causes us to sleep, what occurs during sleep, how our body responds to a lack of sleep and what functions sleep fulfils.

Sleep involves specific cues for its regulation. Sleep is not a passive event, but rather an active process involving characteristic physiological changes in the organs of the body. Sleep is a highly organised sequence of events that follows a regular cyclic program each night.

While there are some modest decreases in metabolic rate during sleep, there's no evidence that any major organ or regulatory system in the body shuts down. Some brain activity increases dramatically and the endocrine system increases secretion of hormones, such as growth hormone. In rapid eye movement (REM) sleep, many parts of the brain are as active as at any time of wakefulness.

When daily sleep time is less than an individual needs, a sleep debt develops. Even small daily reductions in sleep time can accumulate across days to cause a sleep debt. If the debt becomes too great, it can lead to problem sleepiness. Although the individual may not be aware of his or her sleepiness, the sleep debt can have powerful effects on daytime performance, thinking and mood. Eventually the body requires that the debt be paid.

Eight hours of sleep per night appears to be optimal for most adults, although some may need more or less. Teenagers, on average, require about nine or more hours of sleep per night to be as alert as possible when awake.

It doesn't appear that we're able to adapt to getting less sleep than our body requires. In addition to its myriad detrimental effects on health, lack of sleep can also make us fat. That's right — besides impaired recovery and repair, and decreased secretion of growth hormone, sleep deprivation can cause elevated levels of cortisol (a stress hormone), which influences our blood sugar and increases our risk of excess fat deposition.

I've probably just opened a can of worms for the next bestselling book, entitled *Sleep Yourself Slim*!

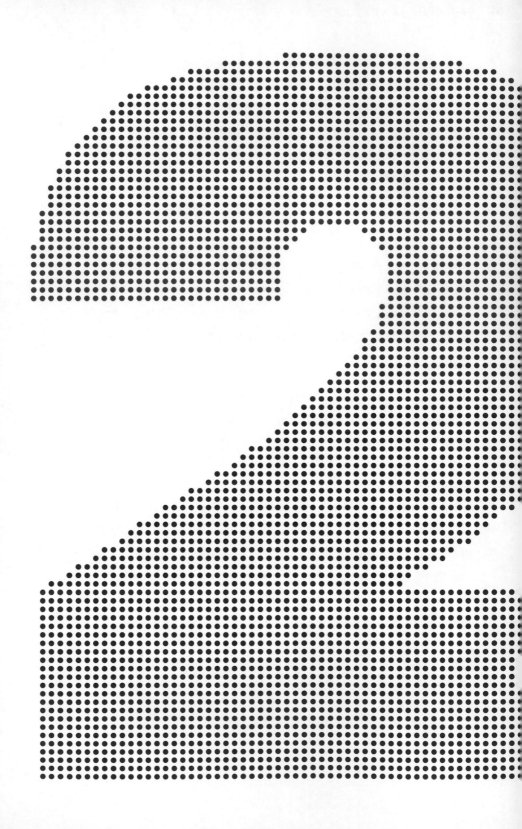

WHAT YOU CAN DO

IT'S UP TO YOU

If you can be sufficiently open-minded to try a change — and for many of you it's probably a radical change — you'll find yourself pleasantly surprised. Whether your goal is to trim some body fat, increase strength or endurance, or take control of ailments such as diabetes or high cholesterol, *it's up to you*. Remember, this is not something you do for six weeks to lose 6 kilos. It's a real commitment you are making to yourself and you will need to remind yourself of this each day until it becomes second nature.

The exhilaration of getting your body into shape is uniquely exciting, rewarding and challenging. It can almost feel miraculous, as though you have become a champion in a battle that, for many years, seemed too fierce to even enter. Enjoy!

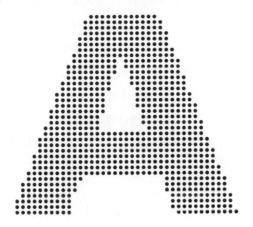

DIET

While exercise is an important part of getting your body into shape and keeping it there, the food you choose to eat is the single most important factor when it comes to permanent fat loss.

TOO MUCH OF A GOOD THING

If the first challenge is fine-tuning your palate to the pleasures of clean, healthy food, the second challenge is regulating the quantities of good food you consume. Too much of a good thing can still be detrimental to health. Even excessive amounts of healthy food will be stored by the body as fat.

You may have corrected the food balance so that your diet is a well-measured variety of protein, colourful plant foods and good fats, but too much and your weight will increase. There is such a thing as too many salads, healthy shakes or fruit. Watch the volume.

One of the primary reasons for excess weight gain is an energy imbalance, where the calories consumed exceed the calories expended. Filling up on low-sugar, low-calorie goodies will still show up on the hips if the overall quantities exceed your requirements.

Food portions are crucial in balancing those scales and correcting the dreaded plateau that so often strikes when the weight refuses to budge. If you want 24 per cent body fat but remain stuck at 30 per cent, it's because you're eating and exercising in the way someone of 30 per cent body fat would. Change and your body will change with you.

Trim the portions, rectify the protein–carbohydrate balance or tweak your training regimen so that you burn more calories, and the plateau will invariably shift and the fat will budge while you're still eating plenty of good foods.

HYPOTHETICAL #2

THE PROBLEM

Greg is a workaholic — a dilemma close to my heart. He's up before dawn and is rarely home before dusk. Much of the day is spent in meetings (with typical 'white sandwich' catering), on a plane or buried under mountains of paperwork at his desk. The vending machine is his friend, as is the staff-room biscuit tin. He's gained a substantial amount of weight around his belly in recent years and has now been advised by his doctor to lose at least 15 kilos for health reasons. Both time restrictions and the logistics of changing his food and fitting in exercise are proving to be a problem.

THE SOLUTION

DIET

Time management and priority.

» On his way into the office, Greg should drop in to the local cafe to place an order for his lunch. This takes around sixty seconds, as does picking it up at lunchtime — probably the same amount of time it takes to put coins in the slot of the vending machine.

» Grab a couple of pieces of fruit from home and have them at the office to appease 'biscuit o'clock'.

» Have a substantial breakfast. This is very important. It will set Greg up for the day and help curb the four o'clock munchies. Prepare something the night before. If it means getting up five minutes earlier to eat it, so be it.

» Never skip breakfast. Even if it means grabbing a couple of hard-boiled eggs and an apple from the fridge as he runs out of the house, Greg has no excuse for skipping breakfast. These bad habits will only set him up for a blood-sugar roller-coaster ride and consequent cravings.

» Don't go to meetings hungry. If this is unavoidable, Greg may be able to have a say in the catering to ensure he'll have some healthy choices.

» Drink at least 2 litres of water a day and cut back on coffee. Avoid milk and sugar in tea or coffee. Be wary of high-calorie beverages such as hot chocolate, frappuccinos, mochachinos (or any 'chino', for that matter) and chai lattes.

» When dining out, Greg needs to ask for exactly what he wants to eat. Don't settle for 'however it comes'. Nobody thinks twice these days about making little changes to menu items, such as sauces on the side or changing a side dish from fries to a salad. Greg needs to ensure the meal includes a large salad or serving of vegetables to fill him up and stop him from reaching for the fluffy white dinner rolls.

STRENGTH

It all boils down to his trusty BlackBerry!

» He should book training in as an appointment at least three times a week and give it the same priority as he would any other 'meeting'.

» If Greg needs to be accountable, I recommend a recurring booking with a personal trainer. If he struggles with time, he can find a trainer who'll come to him. Many people need a trainer to drag them by the ear from behind their desks. Believe me, I've done it. These days, I've organised for a trainer to do this to me!

» Travel is not an excuse to miss training. Hotels all have gyms — and personal trainers.

» If Greg's not keen on going to the gym, he can follow a simple routine of 100 repetitions of exercise every day. For example, twenty push-ups, twenty sit-ups, twenty squats, twenty burpees and twenty tricep dips off a chair. If he does this religiously each day before his morning shower, Greg will find this is a great way to improve muscle tone and strength in only five to ten minutes a day. No time commitment, no additional travel or expense … no excuses!

CARDIO

Twenty to thirty minutes a day — every day.

» For Greg it would be ideal to have a walk or run before his day begins. There's no doubt his day would run away from him if he tried to exercise after work. Besides getting it out of the way early, he'd feel energetic and alert all day long. Greg could find a buddy or work colleague to join him, and this may help him to stay on track. And there's nothing like a bit of competition in the workplace to fuel motivation.

» If running isn't Greg's thing, he could try an early-morning bike ride with a mate or even hiring a stationary cycle to use in the comfort of his own home. Greg could wake up and jump straight on his bike to catch the 6 am news bulletin, with his exercise for the day completed by 6.30.

SMART FAT LOSS

'What, when and how much should I eat?' This is the most popular question I'm asked on a daily basis; from novice to athlete the dilemma is the same. Of course the answer depends greatly on your lifestyle, your likes and dislikes, where you live, how active you are, what your body composition is, as well as what your goals are and any food intolerances or allergies you have.

The main focus for individuals of all fitness levels is to balance blood sugar. It seems like a simple plan, but even with the amount of foods that are available today, many of us still have a tough time implementing this with any consistency. But don't despair — I have devised a very simple plan for navigating your road to optimal health, fat loss and energy.

I like to teach my clients about their hunger, and eating when they know their bodies need food rather than eating from habit or relying on the clock. Blood glucose will rise and fall throughout the day, so while it's important to eat regularly, it's imperative to identify the hunger response and learn to listen to your body. But it's difficult to do this if the foods you're choosing to eat are causing dramatic blood-sugar fluctuations.

By using a few basic nutrition facts, balancing your blood sugar becomes much easier than you may think. Manipulating macronutrients (protein, carbohydrates and fats) can keep cravings at bay and help you stay fuller for longer. This will also better regulate blood-sugar levels and provide a consistent amount of energy, thus avoiding the dreaded three o'clock munchies. Once this is under control you'll no longer be tempted to dig your mitts into the office biscuit tin, or knock someone out of the way to get to the pantry the minute you get home.

Rather than focusing solely on calorie intake, manipulation of macronutrients ensures that lean protein, healthy fat and unprocessed carbohydrates are eaten at each main meal. The combination of the protein, fat and unprocessed carbs will not only provide an excellent concentration of nutrients, but it will effectively stabilise your blood sugar. This will leave you feeling fuller for longer and can also improve blood fats, health, energy levels and body composition.

Putting this into action is a piece of cake (if you'll pardon the expression). The modular food plan detailed in this book will help you to accurately manipulate your nutrient intake for optimum fat loss, energy and overall health. It's as simple as choosing three main meals and an optional two snacks per day. Your precise portion sizes are also detailed in this plan to allow you to then personalise it. The closer you stick to this, the faster your fat loss will be.

What I'm proposing are effective dietary habits for a lifetime. No calorie counting, loads of variety, the freedom to choose the foods you like and maximum fat loss. This formula in itself will regulate your blood sugar beautifully and, consequently, help you to lose fat faster and more effectively than ever before.

THE 'x 100' PRINCIPLE

Take your current weight and multiply it by 100 to calculate how many kilojoules you currently consume each day to sustain where you are.

If you'd like to lose weight, simply choose your goal weight on the chart and you'll instantly know how many kilojoules you need to eliminate. Simple!

As you will now know from previous chapters, your body is a mirror image of your lifestyle, so I've created a chart to make this system easy to use and understand. The column on the left lists various weights. On the right you will see how many kilojoules or calories it takes to maintain each weight.

How does this work for you? Well, if you are currently 90 kilos

WEIGHT IN KILOGRAMS	SUPPORT KILOJOULES/CALORIES*
50	5000/1196
55	5500/1316
60	6000/1435
65	6500/1555
70	7000/1675
75	7500/1794
80	8000/1914
85	8500/2033
90	9000/2153
95	9500/2273
100	10,000/2392
105	10,500/2512
110	11,000/2632
115	11,500/2751
120	12,000/2871

*kilojoules/calories required to support/maintain
a specific weight on the scales

OPTIMUM FAT LOSS = GOAL WEIGHT x 100

FOR EXAMPLE:

CURRENT WEIGHT x 100	**= 90 KILOS** = 9000 KJ/2153 CALORIES
GOAL WEIGHT x 100	**= 60 KILOS** = 6000 KJ/1435 CALORIES
OVERCONSUMING/ UNDEREXERCISING	*= 3000 KJ/718 CALORIES*

and you wish to get down to 60 kilos, you'll see that you are overconsuming/underexercising by an average of 3000 kJ or 718 calories a day. Now that we know the scope of the problem, we have a much better chance of fixing it — no more wasting time guessing and getting it wrong, or trying to follow a 'one size fits all' program.

This shows you are in 'surplus' of 3000 kJ per day, so to shed 30 kilos of fat you must reduce your food intake and increase your exercise to wipe off 3000 kJ (718 calories) each day to return to your healthy weight.

If you are 'calorie literate' you can go ahead and use this vital information to accurately map out your food choices. If you find calorie counting monotonous (as most of us do), just refer to the detailed menu planner (on page 102-08). Simply find the category of your *goal* weight and begin to follow the plan. Eat and exercise as you would at your goal weight and your body will have no choice but to follow you there.

These excess kilojoules can be burned in extra activity, by reducing your food intake, or a combination of both. My preference, and the most sustainable option, is the last. You will need to look at the amount of time you have to dedicate to exercise and lock this into your diary. Anything over and above this will have to be adapted through your food choices. To help you decide what percentage of your excess you

EXERCISE	APPROXIMATE CALORIES BURNED/HOUR	APPROXIMATE KILOJOULES BURNED/HOUR
WALKING (6–7KM/H)	300	1254
JOGGING (9–10KM/H)	500	2090
JUMPING ROPE (100+ JUMPS PER MINUTE)	650	2717
SWIMMING (MODERATE PACE)	300	1254
WEIGHT TRAINING (MODERATE INTENSITY/PACE)	450	1881
CYCLING (MODERATE PACE)	300	1254
TENNIS (SINGLES)	350	1463

need to burn off in activity, I've calculated a chart for you.

If you have a 700 calorie (2926 kJ) daily surplus to eliminate, it would be very difficult and time consuming to spend more than two hours a day trying to walk it off. In this case, the most sustainable option would be a 30:70 ratio: 30 per cent exercise and 70 per cent diet. For example: burn 210 calories more through a forty-minute walk, and eat 490 fewer calories by eliminating two caffè lattes and your afternoon chocolate hit.

I hope this gives you some perspective on the influence your body composition and activity can have on the amount of food you can eat. If you choose to be sedentary for much of the day, you will have to adjust your food intake to be as close to your BMR as possible to avoid excess fat gain. The more active you are, the broader the buffer zone you'll have.

MODULAR MENU PLANNER

GROUP ONE
MAIN MEALS

	F1 — Female Goal weight 55–60 kg [54 kg or less -25% from quantities]	F2 — Female Goal weight 61–66 kg [67 kg or more +25% to quantities]	M1 — Male Goal weight 73–78 kg [72 kg or less -25% from quantities]	M2 — Male Goal weight 79–85 kg [...ore +25% to quantities]
OMELETTE				
Whole egg	0	1	2	3
Egg white	5	5	6	6
Cheese	20 g	30 g	50 g	80 g
Spinach, tomato, mushroom, etc.	unlimited	unlimited	unlimited	unlimited
MUESLI				
Homemade/raw muesli without dried fruit	½ cup	¾ cup	1 cup	1½ cups
Whey Protein Isolate powder (WPI)	30 g	40 g	50 g	60 g
Natural yoghurt or reduced-fat milk	100 g/mL	150 g/mL	200 g/mL	250 g/mL
Fresh or frozen berries	small handful (80 g)	small handful (100 g)	handful (150 g)	handful (180 g)

PORRIDGE

Rolled oats	30 g	40 g	60 g	80 g
Whey Protein Isolate powder (WPI)	30 g	40 g	50 g	60 g
Water	as required	as required	as required	as required
Reduced-fat milk	n/a	100 mL	200 mL	250 mL
Fresh or frozen berries	small handful (80 g)	small handful (100 g)	handful (150 g)	handful (180 g)

SHAKE

Frozen berries or cherries	100 g	100 g	150 g	200 g
Whey Protein Isolate powder (WPI)	30 g	40 g	50 g	60 g
Water	as required	as required	as required	as required
Reduced-fat milk	100 mL (optional)	150 mL (optional)	200 mL	250 mL
Flaxseed oil	2 teaspoons	2 teaspoons	3 teaspoons	3 teaspoons

POACHED EGGS

Eggs	2	2	3	4
Smoked salmon	50 g	75 g	150 g	200 g
Spinach	unlimited	unlimited	unlimited	unlimited
Avocado	¼	½	¾	1
Tomato	1	1	2	2

GROUP ONE
MAIN MEALS

	F1	F2	M1	M2
FRUIT & YOGHURT				
Natural (unflavoured) yoghurt	100 g	150 g	200 g	250 g
Whey Protein Isolate powder (WPI)	30 g	40 g	50 g	60 g
Berries, any variety	100 g	150 g	200 g	250 g
Crushed raw nuts, any variety	20 g	30 g	50 g	70 g
CHICKEN & AVOCADO SALAD				
Cooked skinless chicken breast	80 g	100 g	150 g	200 g
Avocado	¼	½	1	1½
Cheese, feta or hard variety	30 g	40 g	50 g	60 g
Cherry tomatoes	4	6	8	8
Green leaves and additional vegetables, such as peppers, mangetout and green beans	unlimited	unlimited	unlimited	unlimited
BEEF STIR-FRY				
Lean eye fillet steak	raw weight 100 g	raw weight 130 g	raw weight 180 g	raw weight 250 g
Assorted colourful vegetables, such as baby bok choy, mange tout, peppers, Chinese cabbage, fresh ginger, fresh chillies	2 cups	2½ cups	3 cups	4 cups
Tamari sauce to taste				

FISH & ASIAN GREENS

Fresh fish (tuna, salmon, etc)

Chicken stock (optional)

Fresh herbs and spices to taste

	raw weight 100 g	raw weight 130 g	raw weight 180 g	raw weight 250 g
Assorted Asian green vegetables and fresh bean shoots	2 cups	3 cups	4 cups	4 cups

HOMEMADE CHICKEN SOUP

Made fresh with skinless chicken breast, unlimited 'starchy' colourful vegetables, stock and fresh herbs and spices

(This can be frozen in serving sizes and heated up as required.)

cooked volume 1 cup (250 ml) incl. approx 80 g chicken/serve	cooked volume 1½ cups (375 mL) incl. approx. 100 g chicken/serve	cooked volume 2 cups (500 mL) incl. approx. 150 g chicken/serve	cooked volume 3 cups (750 mL) incl. approx. 200 g chicken/serve

SALAD NICOISE

Tuna (cooked fresh or tinned in water)

	cooked weight 80 g	cooked weight 100 g	cooked weight 150 g	cooked weight 200 g
Hard-boiled egg	1	1½	2	3
Olives	4	6	8	8
Leaves, green beans	1 cup	1½ cups	2 cups	2½ cups
Anchovies (optional)	2	3	4	5

Drizzle with balsamic vinegar and sprinkle with cracked pepper and fresh herbs.

GROUP ONE
MAIN MEALS

	F1	F2	M1	M2
QUICK & EASY BARBECUED CHICKEN				
Barbecued chicken, no skin	cooked weight 80 g	cooked weight 100 g	cooked weight 150 g	cooked weight 200 g
Pre-packaged coleslaw mix	1 cup	1½ cups	2 cups	3 cups
Dressing: small amount of low-cal mayo diluted with fresh lemon juice	1 dessertspoon	1 dessertspoon	1½ dessertspoons	2 dessertspoons
BAKED FISH PARCELS				
Fresh fish fillet, any variety, topped with desired herbs and spices or slices of lemon and seasoning. Wrap in a foil parcel lined with waxed paper and bake in a moderate oven for approximately twenty minutes or until cooked through.	raw weight 100 g	raw weight 130 g	raw weight 180 g	raw weight 250 g
Salad greens	1 cup	1½ cups	2 cups	3 cups
Dressing: low-cal French dressing	1 teaspoon	1 teaspoon	2 teaspoons	3 teaspoons
STEAK				
Lean cut of rib eye fillet, grilled, seasoned with sea salt and pepper	raw weight 100 g	raw weight 130 g	raw weight 180 g	raw weight 250 g
Rocket	1 cup	1½ cups	2 cups	2 cups
Shaved parmesan	20 g	30 g	40 g	50 g
Dressing: lemon juice and vinegar to taste				

GROUP TWO
SNACKS

FRUIT & CHEESE

Finely sliced, good-quality hard cheese, such as Parmesan or Swiss	20 g	30 g	50 g	70 g
Finely sliced fresh fruit, such as apple or pear	1 small piece fruit	1 small piece fruit	1 medium piece fruit	1 large piece fruit

Serve the cheese on the sliced fruit.

RAW NUTS

Any variety, raw and unsalted	20 g	30 g	50 g	75 g

APPROVED PROTEIN BAR

See www.DonnaAston.com for details	30 g	30 g	60 g	60 g

VEGIE STICKS & DIP

Vegies such as carrot, celery and cucumber	unlimited	unlimited	unlimited	unlimited

GROUP TWO
SNACKS

	F1	F2	M1	M2
'DIP' MADE FROM:				
hard-boiled eggs	1	1	2	3
low-cal mayo	½ teaspoon	½ teaspoon	1 teaspoon	1 teaspoon
avocado	¼ small	½ small	1 medium	1 large
Tabasco and seasoning, to taste				
TOMATO & CHEESE				
Ripe plum tomatoes, thickly sliced	1 whole.	1 whole	2 whole	2 whole
Cheese, any variety	30 g	40 g	50 g	60 g
Sea salt, cracked pepper				
FUDGE BALLS				
Recipe in *Fat or Fiction*	2	3	4	5

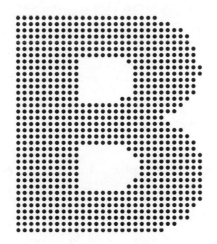

HABITS

LEARNING TO **APPLY THE BRAKES**

If you've stuck to healthy living, you don't *deserve* to eat a box of Smarties, you deserve to stay healthy. Being good is not a hobby that should be rewarded by being bad; just be smart.

Many years ago, when I changed my personal approach to food, I not only lost all physical yearning to ever break out and have chocolate but, after a while, eating poorly actually made me feel ill. I call it a 'food hangover'. I may as well drink a bottle of vodka as eat chocolate, I feel just as unwell the following day. I have maintained such a clean diet for so many years that I need no more convincing than the signals from my own body. I don't want headaches, fatigue or nausea. I can't afford to feel anything less than 100 per cent and I make sure I never do.

Having said this, I don't expect you to be 'perfect'. If you aim too high, you will fail every time. This is a real problem for many. You know the drill. You try to stick to a regimented plan each day, but … a catered all-day meeting is called at the office, you're invited to a friend's place for a big pasta meal, it's your boss's birthday drinks after work, and so on. This is life. Shit happens! If you try to be perfect through each and every one of these scenarios you will either have to become a social hermit or be ribbed by your colleagues and friends for bringing your little red plastic lunchbox to every occasion. The alternative that many take in these situations is to throw caution to the wind and bin the diet. Many of us have an all-or-nothing approach. All rational thought and logic seems to go out the window when it comes to food.

We need to find a happy medium and know when to stop justifying the 'sneaky treats' and apply the brakes. So what do you do in those awkward situations? Just do the best you can. If you're served a meal that doesn't really work for you, just pick around it, resisting the fluffy white dinner roll and the crème brûlée. In other work-based situations, think ahead and bring a snack where it's appropriate. Ditto when you're travelling. Enjoy the celebratory drinks but slow down and alternate alcohol with water. You can live quite comfortably — and slimly — like this for the long haul.

Remember, having that chocolate bar on a *regular* basis can set you back. Apart from unsettling your digestive balance, the 'it won't hurt' approach is an attitude that becomes cumulative and begins to justify some bad habits. If you think that you got away with it once or twice, it's human nature to test the boundaries. Before long the weight is back, and then some, and you have to start all over again.

The super model Kate Moss once said, 'Nothing tastes as good as skinny feels.' A far better version is, 'Nothing tastes as good as *healthy* feels.'

MY TIPS FOR STAYING ON TRACK:

» It's crucial to keep setting 'stepping stone' goals so achievements are attainable and measurable.

» Keep challenging yourself so you're reminded that it wasn't easy to lose that weight, and to keep good health exciting and rewarding. Aim to jog a certain distance without stopping, build up to skipping 180 jumps a minute, enter a fun run, or set about improving strength or tone in specific areas.

» Establish a six- or twelve-month planner to keep on track and revise it whenever you reach a landmark. Staying fit and well doesn't stop once you reach a goal — it's a way of life and a euphoric work in progress.

» Some will say, 'You've got to live,' and I couldn't agree more. But you need to decide whether 'living' means enjoying five-minute taste sensations and having an overfat, lethargic body, or enjoying a lifelong, life-enhancing, life-extending journey in a great body.

The 'secret' to weight control is to value yourself enough to follow a program for the rest of your life that will maintain a healthy, disease-free body and optimum quality of life.

Oh, and remember: it's much easier to keep it off than to lose it all over again … and again … and again.

STOP TRYING TO
OUTSMART YOUR BODY

The world of breakfast-phobes is fascinating, filled with misinformation and peculiar constraints.

Scared to eat in the morning, rising with an iron will they tell themselves it's too early to eat. They have no appetite and, besides, breakfast will only make them gain weight, right?

The result of such restraint is that by mid-morning they're ravenous and by 4 pm it's all over. The vending machine at the office has never looked so appealing, with chocolates, biscuits and snacks coming at a fast and furious pace, only to be topped up with dinner a few hours later. Going to bed without any hunger but with an overly satiated stomach is comforting for some. Unfortunately, this habit of filling up late in the day starts the 'not hungry for breakfast' cycle all over again the next morning. It's like Groundhog Day!

Even those who like breakfast start small, 'saving' themselves for the best and biggest meal of the day — dinner. Calorie restriction is metered out until the 'real' meal at the end of the day. The problem with this pattern is that it's likely to lead to weight gain and is certainly prohibitive to weight loss.

We actually need to eat a certain amount of food throughout the day. If you've only eaten one-third of the required amount of food before dinner that means you're eating the bulk at night when activity is at a minimum.

All eating should be completed two to three hours before going to bed because this allows food to leave the stomach and enter the digestive tract. Digestion slows right down once you're asleep so it's not advisable to have food in the stomach when you go to bed.

But I'm not suggesting you graze throughout the day. I'm not a great fan of constant snacking and personally I only eat three meals a day. I rarely snack; if I know I'll be eating at an irregular time I'll have an apple, but I can usually organise my life to avoid this as well. I'm a big believer in all meals having a start and, most importantly, an end.

People talk about grazing to maintain a high metabolism but the extra calories consumed tend to far outweigh any metabolic increase. Much of the obsession people develop for food is because they are always thinking, 'What's next?' They have breakfast and think of their mid-morning snack; they have lunch and think of afternoon tea, and at dinner they think of supper or a little treat before bed. The world becomes about food, giving it an importance that cannot realistically be maintained in the long term.

Breakfast, lunch and dinner, yes. And try not to save all your calories until the end of the day. Distribute them throughout those three meals, or even try shifting the balance to the earlier meals: your weight will benefit as much as your energy levels and your health. That old adage is so true: breakfast like a king, lunch like a prince (or princess) and dine like a pauper.

CHANGING **LIFELONG HABITS**

Say you want to create a new habit, whether it's taking more exercise, eating more healthily or both. How often does it need to be performed before it no longer requires superhuman self-control?

Google it and you'll likely find a figure of twenty-one days. In fact, there's no solid evidence for this number at all. It's thought that this figure may have originated from a book published in 1960 by a plastic surgeon. Dr Maxwell Maltz noticed that amputees took an average of twenty-one days to adjust to the loss of a limb, so he argued that people take twenty-one days to adjust to any major life changes. Unless you get hungry enough to chew your own arm off, this may not be particularly relevant.

I think the process of changing diet and exercise habits is not unlike quitting smoking: it may take more than one try. You may have a rational justification for why you also couldn't make it work on the second or third try. And then, finally, it may suddenly kick in on the tenth attempt. You could admit defeat after the fourth or fifth attempt, but instead, persevere, learn from each experience — never quit quitting those bad habits — and you'll get there in the end.

It takes conscious effort to change everyday lifestyle habits, which are generally dealt with on a subconscious level. Take it one day at a time, be patient with yourself, don't allow a few slip-ups to throw you completely off track and you'll succeed in the end. If you continue to look at these experiences as failures rather than learning experiences, you'll place a very negative slant on the process, making it increasingly difficult to succeed. Thomas Edison was once asked if he was discouraged by his 10,000 failed attempts to invent a commercially viable incandescent light bulb before he eventually succeeded. He famously responded, 'I have not failed. I've just found 10,000 ways that won't work.'

KNOWING **YOUR ABC**

A wise psychology professor once taught me a great tool I often use to try to change bad habits or negative behaviour. The ABC method can be applied to any negative situation or obstacle you wish to change to a more positive outcome.

The letter A is for Activating an event. It can relate to an internal thought or an external event. For example, you've joined a new gym and you're going for your first workout tonight.

The letter B is for Belief. This is your belief or thought process about the event. For example, every time you go to the gym you feel uncomfortable and really unfit and uncoordinated.

The letter C is for emotional Consequence. This is the emotion you feel due to your interpretation or belief. For example, you have now been overcome by unjustified, irrational negative feelings about something that has not yet taken place.

So how can you change this? It's all about being aware of this negative process and catching yourself when you start to do it. Once you identify the flaw in your thinking, you can use this model to replace your belief with a more positive thought. For the purpose of the gym example above, if your belief is that you're excited about your first step towards a healthier, fitter you, your emotions before you arrive and the experience you have when you start will be completely different. It's a gradual conditioning exercise, but once you're aware of it you'll be amazed at how many times you catch yourself with negative beliefs that are likely to sabotage your weight-loss efforts time and again.

MY TIPS:

»   Practise your ABCs.

»   Keep it positive. Rather than telling yourself: 'I must get rid of this flab', think; 'I want to be lean, fit and strong.'

»   Change your routines. If you've identified a particularly difficult time of day when your eating habits are poor, create a new pattern to avoid this situation.

»   Be prepared for people who may sabotage your change. Be assertive and tell them why this is detrimental to your efforts.

»   Accept the occasional relapse. If you can treat it as nothing more than a slight slip that teaches you something, then you're on the right track.

ARE YOUR EYES BIGGER
THAN YOUR STOMACH?

We're all taught to save for a rainy day, to take a jacket just in case it gets cold, to never leave the house without lipstick in case we have an accident. Much of the behaviour we're raised with is preparatory, and our eating habits are more of the same.

Remember how our mothers packed our lunchboxes with more food than we could ever eat, in case we were hungry at school? Most of us would usually take at least one lunchbox item home from school every day — usually the banana — and our mothers would do a daily inventory. We'd always receive praise if we'd polished off the lot. The same process took place again during the evening meal, when you had to finish every last scrap from your plate or you wouldn't be given dessert. This theory of completion at all costs leads to non-hungry eating, over-formalised eating patterns and often excess weight.

Fear of hunger is one of the most instinctive human responses. It's understandable in developing nations but I hear so many people from affluent societies talk anxiously about getting hungry as though it is such a terror that it's worth going to extreme lengths to prevent it.

Our fear of hunger seems only to be relieved by overeating, usually at lunch or dinner, just in case hunger pounces later in the day and we find ourselves stranded on a desert island (in one of our huge metropolitan cities) with nothing to eat. The primal survival urge of hunger is designed to signal to us when we require sustenance. Through conditioning, often in our childhood, this signal becomes distorted or even irrelevant when it comes to regulating appetite.

Feeling hungry actually means the body is working efficiently; the flip side is when the stomach is full to the brim, causing digestion to be uncomfortable and inefficient. Add to this the consumption of overprocessed foods and wild blood-sugar fluctuations and we have created a sensory minefield.

If we truly listened more to our bodies, our appetites could be better managed. Confront the fear of getting hungry and recognise that there's a difference between being full and being satisfied. It is much more comfortable to be satisfied and still have room to move rather than to flop on the couch with a bloated body, feeling stodgy and remorseful. It's also important to remember that it can take twenty to thirty minutes after eating for your brain to register that your stomach is full. For this reason, it's important to ensure you eat slowly and chew your food well. Gone are the days when you inhale your meal and head to the kitchen in search of seconds, only to find yourself thirty minutes later feeling like you may burst. Sit, relax, chew, enjoy.

For women, hormones will affect the appetite at certain times of the month, making it either insatiable or nonexistent (commonly the former). Certain foods work brilliantly to keep hunger at bay: foods that are high in protein keep you feeling fuller for longer, so the body is well nourished and fuelled when it has meat, nuts, cheese, pulses or yoghurt to work with. Keeping well hydrated by drinking pure water is also very important when it comes to controlling appetite. On the other hand, high-carbohydrate foods will upset blood sugar, leading to cravings for more of those foods and exacerbating hunger as well as providing poor nutrition. Most people are amazed when they lose all taste or yearning for chocolate or bread once they switch the balance of their diet to include more lean protein and fresh plant foods and fewer processed carbs. Their hunger also levels out.

We all know appetite is often emotional rather than physical. People tend to eat for comfort and reassurance, or out of boredom, stress or even anger. The greater the emotional needs, the greater the appetite. Regardless, emotional eating often doesn't provide relief. It is really worth thinking about your appetite and listening to your body. It may not be as hungry as you think it is.

TIPS TO KEEP PORTIONS UNDER CONTROL:

» Eat only at the table. Don't do a *Seinfeld* and eat straight from the pantry or the fridge.

» Don't pick from your children's meals or feel compelled to clear their plates for them. If they're sensible enough to know when they're full, then maybe your own clean plate means you have had enough too. Contrary to popular belief, there is no need to force kids, or yourself, to finish eating everything on the plate.

» Downsize the dinner plate and only eat what you serve yourself. Don't be tempted to have a second (or fifth) helping.

» Take time to eat and enjoy your meals by chewing properly and savouring all the flavours. It generally takes around twenty to thirty minutes for your stomach to signal to your brain that you're full. Remember this when you go hunting around the kitchen immediately after dinner.

» Don't eat for stress relief because you will never be satiated. Eating does not alleviate stress, and can often make it worse. Emotional or comfort eating tends to mean overeating.

» Relax before you eat by walking or exercising. It prepares your body to be refuelled.

» Never abstain from eating so much that you become ravenous. Starvation brings on panic and you will eat anything in sight. Temper your appetite by thinking ahead and having a few healthy snacks readily available in case you need them.

» Always ensure the nutritional balance is met in your meals so there's enough protein, vegetables (at least five to seven portions a day) and good fats, which also keep hunger at bay.

FAD ADDICTION

There is a big secret to weight loss.

It's not to stop eating at 3 pm, to only sip soup or to have your blood tested to discover which foods you should avoid.

It's not that complicated. As more of us struggle with our weight and we're eating more on the run, shrewd marketing companies see the opportunity to pounce on our vulnerability with that elusive quick fix.

But there is only one way to lose weight. The great secret is to become more conscious of food choices and to move more. It may not sound as exciting as the Blood Type Diet or Atkins or the Zone but it is the truth. The great *deception* comes in many guises and is always billed as a 'new diet'. Sometimes it costs a lot of money and requires counting, reading and doing lots of sums.

It is always the answer everyone has been looking for when other weight-loss methods have failed.

People wanting to lose weight tend to be defenceless against falling for the latest thing, as though something external will make them lose weight rather than them working to shift their psychology and their whole approach to life.

Trying a new approach is understandable and can be a great source of motivation, especially when the new diet fads mostly come with guarantees of quick results. But being a fad addict can also be a way of avoiding reality.

No matter how it's packaged, the message of every diet is to reduce your calories, to think about what you are eating and to get the most nutritional value from your food.

It takes time. You don't gain 3 kilos in a week, so you can't expect to lose fat at that rate. Losing body fat in a healthy way doesn't happen quickly, so the motivation comes by taking small steps — for the rest of your life. Stop looking for a six-week wonder and accept that you need to make positive changes for an everyday wonder that will change your life.

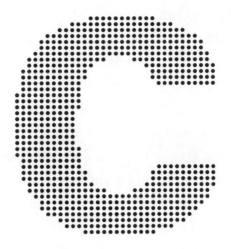

EXERCISE

WHEN DOES EXERCISE **BECOME FUN?**

For those of us who spent our childhood praying for rain or illness to get out of PE classes at school, exercise wasn't only unpleasant, it was traumatic. I know, I was one of them.

Watching the vault and the gym mats being prepared in the assembly hall meant the dreaded gym class was unavoidable. The only answer was to hide in the toilets or run to the sick bay, where the kindly nurse could always find something wrong with you and take pity. It's little surprise then that when exercise becomes non-compulsory those of us who spent our childhood avoiding anything other than skipping rope and hopscotch always choose to avoid it.

Ball games continue to terrify us, automatically causing our bodies to leap in the opposite direction of any ball that comes hurtling towards us. Swimming brings back memories of furious instructors too used to yelling at unruly children.

When the weight starts piling on, the mind turns to thoughts of the gym: everywhere there are tightly clothed bodies (which seem to know what they're doing), torturous-looking machines, super-fit blondes at reception and all those mats again — terrifying!

Of course, it's a misconception, but then so much about exercise is emotional. Once you get past the front desk and manage to work on some of the equipment, day by day and rep by rep your confidence builds as your muscles ache and the endorphins fly into production. It's an exciting time as this whole new world opens up to you and you start to tell your friends, whose eyes gradually become wider and wider, amazed that you're not only getting up at 6 am but you're also doing push-ups … and enjoying them.

You become an expert, advising anyone who wants to listen about technique, weight loss and remedies for aching muscles. Everyone starts to resent you but you don't care because you're getting fit, maybe for the first time in your life, and they're still snacking on Kit Kats.

What they don't realise is that this is a stage and it passes, like the first flush of new romance, and after a few months you either build up your routine, limit your workouts (because there's always an excuse) or revert to childhood exercise trauma and declare that exercise will always be hell.

Those who stick with it not only reap the health benefits, they also develop a new fascination with their glutes and hamstrings. What is going on in there to make them hurt so much, even after years of training?

The world of exercise continues to be surprising, challenging and rewarding. Okay, it's not always fun but it can't just be discipline and fear that keeps us working out regularly. There must be some pleasure in it, after all.

YOU CAN'T OUT-TRAIN A BAD DIET

Many of us enlist the services of a personal trainer with the expectation that this alone will get us to our goal weight. Having been in this industry for a long time, I am obviously a believer in the benefits of personal training. But if you're under the illusion that a couple of sessions a week (or even a day) are going to single-handedly reduce your body fat, think again!

Quite honestly, exercise alone is rarely a successful way of losing weight. There's no doubt that exercise is one of the best things in the world you can do for your health. It also improves mood, relieves stress and is great for your heart. Recent research shows that it even helps you grow new brain cells. Not to mention the fact that people who exercise regularly have lower risk of cancer, heart disease and diabetes. Strength training improves muscle conditioning, potentially raising your basal metabolic rate (BMR). But weight loss due to exercise alone? Not so much.

Here's the truth: the exercise–weight loss equation is far more complex than we've been led to believe. Let's start with calories. Most people overestimate calories burned during exercise (by a long shot), just as they typically underestimate daily calorie consumption (ditto). One study asked individuals struggling with weight loss to keep diligent food diaries. In a controlled environment, the participants were then fed exactly what they had written down and they all lost weight.

As far as exercise 'self-deception' goes, many years ago I worked with clients at a public gym where there was a line-up of at least a dozen treadmills. Every evening there was a queue to use the third treadmill from the end when others were free. I found this so puzzling that one day I had to ask the obvious question, 'Why this machine?' I still smile when I think of the answer. One girl piped up, saying that more calories were burned on this particular treadmill. Huh? That's right — the formula for estimating calorie burn in this machine had obviously been set a little differently to the others and countless gym members actually believed they were burning more calories on that particular treadmill.

Regardless of the computer read-out on the gym equipment, even high-impact aerobics only uses up 500 to 600 calories an hour; walking at a pace of 6 km/h barely uses 300 calories per hour. I hate to be the bearer of bad news, but you can cancel out the walk with two skinny lattes! I've seen people at the gym walk on a treadmill for thirty minutes and then guzzle down 'energy' drinks that would take a three-hour run to burn off. Plus there's good old-fashioned denial. Ever justified scoffing down an extra helping of dessert because you just worked out? Sorry to burst your bubble, but that's like saying you saved some money by buying your groceries at Costco, so you now have enough change left over for a month-long holiday in Tahiti. Wishful thinking — it just doesn't add up.

While the research is very clear that it's almost impossible to keep weight off unless you exercise regularly, using exercise alone as a weight-loss strategy is a recipe for failure. If you were to improve your diet and not exercise, you would lose weight but eventually your metabolism would slow and you would have to eat like a sparrow to sustain your weight loss. If you were to exercise and not work on your diet, you would likely improve your cardio fitness and possibly gain some lean muscle to speed up your metabolism, but not by enough to really lose much body fat. If you pay attention to both exercise and diet, you'll be well on your way to achieving your goals.

Remember, your food choices equate to around 75 per cent of the fat-loss equation. That's why good trainers have a saying: 'You can't out-train a bad diet.' Eat and exercise like your life depends on it ... because it does.

WHEN MORE IS **NOT ALWAYS BETTER**

Yoga, spin, Pilates, weights, Zumba! ... the list is seemingly endless. We should all be aware of the importance of exercise for improving our health and body, but can we do too much? Absolutely. Let's put things into perspective ...

I'm surrounded by exercise and it will never cease to amaze me how many establishments seem to turn a blind eye to the obsessive exerciser. All gyms have members who have obviously overcommitted themselves to several hours of classes, weight training or pounding away on cardio equipment every day. I recently consulted a young girl who attended four or five spin classes a day (no, that's not a misprint), seven days a week. She was beside herself when she had to give this up for two months due to stress fractures in her femur (thigh bone). This was an inevitable side effect of excessive exercise, yet it hadn't seemed to deter her obsessive urge to return to this punishing regime the minute she was able to crawl, let alone walk!

Many of you will know someone who, no matter whether sick or injured, will turn up to work out, or feel stressed and anxious if unable to. Much of the time the obsessive exerciser is attempting to out-train a poor diet, and we now know that this is never going to happen.

So how much is too much? It's sometimes difficult for exercise enthusiasts to acknowledge that more is not better. Rest and recovery are as important as the exercise itself when you're training for a buff body. In fact, it's highly likely that you'll severely hinder your progress if you overdo it.

During resistance training, such as weight training and body weight exercises, you actually cause tiny micro-tears in muscle fibres. After your workout your body is faced with repairing the damage. In order to facilitate this task successfully, our bodies require both time and the appropriate nutritional intake. If the physical demand on our bodies begins to overtake the amount of recovery we allow it, overtraining results. This condition will proliferate if optimum nutrition is ignored.

So when does our enthusiasm become detrimental to our health? Many people tend to overcompensate for poor dietary habits, often using exercise as a form of purging. In my experience, those with a severely distorted body image can very easily fall into this destructive pattern.

It is certainly not uncommon for people to assume that if they exercise enough, they can 'get away with' poor eating habits. This couldn't be further from the truth. In fact, the nutritional requirements of a person who participates in a physically demanding regime are far greater than those of a sedentary person. For this reason I've never understood the way some professional athletes chow down on sugar-laden junk to 'replenish' their bodies following an event or game. Remember, even if you do manage to burn off the calories contained in junk food, you are feeding empty calories to an already nutrient-starved body, only exacerbating many of the above-mentioned symptoms.

WHAT STEPS CAN WE TAKE TO
AVOID OVEREXERCISING?

» Enthusiasm is great, but you must pace yourself. More is not better and will not necessarily get you there sooner, if it gets you there at all.

» Listen to your body. If you're tired and sore, slow down, rest and treat your body to some good, nutritious food to assist recovery.

» Get seven to nine hours' sleep a night. Remember, lack of sleep is not only stressful, it can hinder fat loss.

» Don't participate in resistance training (which requires extensive muscle recovery) more than three to four times a week, and try to space your workouts evenly throughout the week, e.g. Monday, Wednesday and Friday.

» In between resistance workouts, walking, stretching and gentle yoga are the best choices, encouraging improvements in flexibility and cardiovascular fitness without overtaxing your body.

» Set realistic goals. Don't put yourself under undue pressure. Reshaping your body takes time, consistency and patience. If creating a great body were quick and easy, everyone would have one.

» The more intensely you train, the longer your muscles need to recover. As your fitness level and strength progress, your regime may have to change to accommodate them. For example, you may consider splitting your routine to focus on different muscle groups each session, allowing full recovery of those previously trained.

» Optimum quantities of protein, unprocessed carbohydrates

and essential fats are needed to facilitate full recovery. For instance, your body needs at least 1 gram of protein per kilogram of body weight, spread out over several meals throughout the day.

SYMPTOMS OF **OVERTRAINING**

» Suppressed immune system (recurring colds and viruses)

» Joint deterioration (pain and inflammation)

» Loss of valuable lean muscle tissue (actually reducing our metabolic rate, often resulting in weight gain — the opposite of what we're trying to achieve)

» Increased risk of injury

» Nutritional deficiencies (resulting in a multitude of ailments)

» Hormonal disturbances in women (including temporary disruption to menstrual cycles)

» Reduced strength or energy

» Insomnia

» Irritability, anxiety or depression

» Lack of concentration

» Elevated resting heart rate

» Low core body temperature

» Lack of general zest, strength and motivation

I think we all know the symptoms of underexercising!

SO HOW DO WE GET ACTIVE
FOLLOWING AN INJURY?

If you've experienced a debilitating injury you'll know how it can interfere with your life. One of the most common injuries is a bulging disc. The pain can interfere with sleep and the simplest everyday tasks, and can literally take your breath away — I know, I've been there. While such an injury can be brought under control and managed, trusting that any form of exercise won't trigger a flare-up is really difficult. Of course your exercise regime will need to be carefully designed with your injury in mind. But the good news is that not only is exercise possible, but the right sort can dramatically reduce your risk of further pain and injury.

It's always wise to consult a physiotherapist or sports physician before resuming exercise. If you choose to see a fitness professional for advice and guidance it's also important to ask your physio or sports physician for a letter of referral, containing details of your injury and any relevant instructions. You may have to take a few steps backwards in intensity until your stability improves, but once you develop a foundation of strength it will become far more realistic to avoid further injury, while exercising and in everyday movement.

Obviously the benefits of exercise are vast, from improving sleep, enhancing the immune system, controlling weight, improving cardiovascular function, lifting self-esteem and appearance and extending life. A growing concern among companies worldwide is the loss of productivity due to poor health and the risk of insuring unhealthy employees. As corporations become more demanding on our time, they'll also be forced to implement staff health and fitness programs to insure against employee meltdown.

FOR THE ATHLETE IN ALL OF US

EATING FOR PERFORMANCE

You may not consider yourself to be the next Paula Radcliffe, but perhaps you fancy challenging yourself to participate in an upcoming charity fun run, or just getting stuck into a more vigorous exercise regime. The following information is valuable regardless of your fitness level.

Do we need extra carbs for energy before, during or after exercise? This question causes great debate. The key to improving your energy, strength and body composition is a blend of correct physical, mental and nutrition principles. Eating for health should be the primary focal point for all of us, since a high level of fitness and energy cannot be supported without an optimal level of health. Without proper daily nutrition your exercise sessions will be less effective and recovery will take longer.

By paying special attention to regulating your blood-sugar level throughout the day you'll become more metabolically efficient. This means that your body will be able to use your fat and carbohydrate stores more efficiently. Through proper macronutrient manipulation you can teach your body to use more of its stored fat at higher intensities of exercise. This will reduce your reliance on extra carbohydrates during intense exercise sessions, which, from my experience with numerous athletes, will also reduce the risk of gastrointestinal distress. Metabolic efficiency should be a primary goal for all who wish to undertake a sustainable exercise regime and create a better body.

BEFORE COMPETITION

Whether competing at a high level or taking part as a novice in your first fun run, you should not significantly change your nutrition program prior to an event. The concept of macronutrient manipulation becomes even more crucial and familiar foods should be the focal point without introducing anything new. If it ain't broke, don't fix it!

You should consume the same balance of lean protein, unprocessed carbohydrates and healthy fats before an event. For those with sensitive stomachs, I recommend tapering fibre intake down a couple of days before competition. This means reducing the amount of high-fibre foods such as wholegrains and fruits for this short period. It's important to remember that you must implement a gradual reintroduction of dietary fibre over two or three days following the event.

I am quite often asked about carbohydrate loading one or two nights before a race. The bottom line is that I am not a fan. The simple reason is that it completely alters the eating pattern that you have worked so hard to implement in the build-up to your race season. By introducing a large amount of carbohydrate and displacing protein and fat, blood sugar will be altered and your energy levels will be all over the place — the last thing you want a day or two before the race. Stick with what has worked for you in the months leading up to your event. Don't be swayed by the carb pushers!

DURING COMPETITION

In some races it may be difficult for you to maintain your normal daily eating routine, since protein and fat are more slowly absorbed and may lead to gastrointestinal concerns. In longer endurance events consuming a bit of protein and fat can be beneficial, but in shorter events fluid and electrolytes are the main constituents that should be in your nutrition plan.

HYDRATION

Consume about 100 mL to 300 mL of fluid every fifteen to twenty minutes.

CARBOHYDRATES

Ideally, you want to work on improving your metabolic efficiency throughout the year during normal eating and training times, and depend on this high efficiency of using fats during your race. This will lead to a reduced need for refined carbohydrates that can cause gastrointestinal upset, which is the last thing we want to encounter during an event. Your stored body fat is your reserve fuel tank. Your body burns it perfectly when given the chance. If you're going hard, you will likely burn approximately 1000 calories an hour during intense exercise, such as fast running. There are 7700 calories available for use in every kilogram of stored body fat. This means that a 70-kilo person at a very lean 10 per cent body fat will have over 50,000 calories of stored fat — that's more than fifty hours' worth of fuel on board.

ELECTROLYTES

Contrary to clever marketing campaigns, it is not necessary to down litres of colourful sports drinks after a regular workout at the gym or a walk with a friend. The only time electrolytes need to be replaced is when you exercise for a prolonged period of time at high intensity, causing profuse sweating and fluid loss. This narrows the field down to pretty serious athletes. Current research indicates that consuming 500 to 700 milligrams of sodium per litre of fluid should be adequate for athletes. However, I recommend beginning at a minimum of 800 milligrams per hour and adjusting accordingly based on your sweat rate and environmental conditions. Athletes requiring a large amount of electrolytes will need specific supplements. Look for one with a full electrolyte profile and beware of the high sugar concentration. It can cause gastrointestinal distress (diarrhoea), which in turn dehydrates you even further.

AFTER COMPETITION

It's important to replace fluid, sodium, unprocessed carbs and good fats after a race. Ideally, you should consume these nutrients within sixty minutes of finishing to ensure a rapid nutritional recovery. Simply return to your normal, blood-sugar balancing, metabolically efficient eating plan and enjoy a quick recovery.

PERFORMANCE FACTS

Optimum quantities of high-quality protein, unrefined nutrient-dense carbohydrates and essential fatty acids in the appropriate ratios are essential to sufficiently compensate for an athlete's physical exertion, while enabling access to the most effective energy pathways.

Athletes place great demands on their bodies, both physically and mentally. An extraordinary volume of nutrients is required to fuel optimum performance and recovery. There is no question that an athlete needs replenishment following heavy training or competition.

While confectionery may provide calories and reload glycogen stores, it doesn't replenish the body with the much-needed nutrients it requires for optimum health and recovery. Such processed food products contain refined sugar, food colouring and a multitude of artificial ingredients.

Sugar is poison for physical conditioning and recovery, as demonstrated by the following facts:

» Sugar depletes the body of B vitamins (particularly vitamin B6), which are used to metabolise simple sugars. This nutrient depletion may potentially compromise healthy intestinal flora, digestion and absorption of nutrients.

» Sugar also depletes the body of various nutrients and minerals, including magnesium, potassium and vitamin C, all of which play essential roles in physical performance.

» Excessive consumption of refined carbohydrates can cause constriction of blood vessels, elevation of triglycerides and lower valuable HDL (good cholesterol) levels.

» Sugar consumption can increase inflammation, possibly leading to the slow healing of injuries and autoimmune responses such as arthritis.

» Studies show that sugar can potentially increase the production of free radicals, and therefore damage, by 100 per cent (based on consumption of a 75 gram glucose drink) and causes a fall in vitamin E, a potent antioxidant.

» Sugar requires a lot of water to be absorbed into cells; therefore it can exacerbate dehydration, poor digestion and gastrointestinal upset, particularly after exercise.

» Simple sugars may increase the body's production of adrenaline by up to 400 per cent, which can cause adrenal exhaustion.

» Consumption of refined carbohydrates significantly decreases the capacity of our immune system to engulf and destroy bacteria. Sugar can suppress the activity of white blood cells by up to 50 per cent thirty minutes after ingestion, and this immune system suppression can last for up to six hours.

» Sugar can cause hardening of tissue, including that of the blood vessels, the lungs, connective tissue and the lens of the eyes, and can increase chronic inflammation.

» Excessive sugar may cause joints to become brittle and stiffer through the cross-linking of collagen.

BURNING **FAT FOR FUEL**

There are two primary sources of 'fuel' for exercise: carbohydrates and fats. Carbohydrates are used preferentially by the body in those people who consume a high-carbohydrate diet and in those with low levels of fitness when fat metabolism is underdeveloped.

We store only a very limited amount of carbohydrate in our body, typically in the form of approximately 100 grams of liver glycogen and 250 to 400 grams of muscle glycogen, depending on muscle mass or condition. When we run low on carbohydrates, we fatigue very quickly. When you teach your body to rely on fat for fuel, your combustion of carbohydrates diminishes, thus sparing carbohydrates. When you use more fat as fuel, you generate more energy and your carbohydrate supply lasts longer.

We store a relatively unlimited supply of fat for fuel. Even athletes with body fat as low as 6 per cent would find it impossible to exhaust their fat stores. For example, a person weighing 90 kilos with 6 per cent fat has 5.4 kilos of fat, equivalent to 41,580 calories of energy. Intense exercise will use approximately 1000 calories an hour.

Researchers have shown that after a twelve-week program of high-intensity training, the body's ability to burn fat increases by 41 per cent. This was accompanied by a reduced reliance on carbohydrates as a primary source of fuel (M Houston, 'Energy: the basis of human movement', *Exercise Sport Science Review*, 1998, 26, pp. 287–314).

Glucose (sugar) is a powerful regulator of fat metabolism. The higher the glucose content of the blood, the lower the fat metabolism. High blood-glucose levels are generated from dietary carbohydrates. This effect is associated with insulin, which acts to reduce glucose levels and store fat and protein. In the process insulin directly blocks the removal of fat from fat deposits. These deposits are an important source of fat for exercising muscle. Insulin also inhibits fat burning within the muscle. Therefore increased insulin is considered to be antagonistic to fat combustion during exercise.

A study conducted by the University of Texas and the University of Limburg in the Netherlands found that fat metabolism was substantially reduced for the full forty minutes of exercise after carbohydrate loading. It takes as little as 20 grams of ingested carbohydrate (one apple) to raise insulin levels and reduce fat as fuel. A 600 mL bottle of Powerade provides more than double this amount (47.5 grams of carbs) and a 200-gram tub of Nestlé low-fat yoghurt provides 20 grams of carbohydrate due to added sugars.

FACE OR BUTT:
DO WE HAVE TO SACRIFICE ONE FOR THE OTHER?

THE lollipop weight-loss craze has to be one of the worst of all time. It wasn't a diet of lollipops for breakfast, lunch and dinner but rather different diets that went too far and left celebrities such as Victoria Beckham looking so emaciated that their heads appeared too big for their bodies, like a lollipop on a stick.

We may be able to control what we eat and how we exercise, but where the weight is shed is less manageable. How disheartening to lose weight from your forearms before your thighs or your chest before your waist. For most women, the crucial and most immediate areas to lose weight are hips, thighs and butt (waist to knees). Men's problems tend to be higher up, incorporating abdomen, chest and those all-too-common love handles that hug the lower back. Unfortunately, we can't choose to lose weight from a specific area. It would be like trying to burn off petrol from the left side of your tank.

Among my clients men invariably want a flatter stomach and women want to stop worrying if their bum looks big in their new jeans. At a lunch I attended recently the conversation could have been about the latest news topics, politics, religion, world peace … but no. It was all about stomachs. The eternal lament of the female is how to lose that stomach, especially after having a baby. Try as they might, my lunch companions — dining on fish in beer batter with potato wedges — complained that it was just impossible to flatten their bellies. Or if they did, how could they stop their faces from looking drawn?

We may not be able to control where our weight drops but we can be smarter about it. By being smarter about what we eat, we can be healthy *and* avoid the lollipop look. It's about thinking of the whole body, not just specific areas.

Genetics and hormones influence the quantity of fat cells, or storage tanks, that accumulate in specific areas. Yet we remain in control: we can fill them up until they overflow, or we can keep them at a functional, healthy level.

Changing body composition so that lean weight is higher and the body fat is reduced will increase muscle tone beneath the skin, counteracting the drawn look. An overall body fat reduction will reduce all fat stores. The genetically thicker areas where more fat cells accumulate will take longer to reduce but there's no such thing as spot reduction. Doing 100 sit-ups a day won't give you a flat stomach. Abdominal exercises will firm the muscle and improve the underlying shape but achieving a well-balanced and proportioned shape is still going to be about overall body composition.

As we age we do lose some of the fat padding beneath the skin on our faces, just as fat tends to migrate to our hips and waistlines, so there's a fine balance to maintain. A body composition of between 20 per cent and 25 per cent for women and less than 20 per cent for men will usually ensure this balance. Anything lower than 20 per cent body fat for women will probably cause a harder, more angular look to a woman's face and body. More than 30 per cent body fat is not only unhealthy, but you will unlikely be happy with the appearance of it either.

There is no need to be a lollipop. Think muscle and lean weight, then tone will overtake bone.

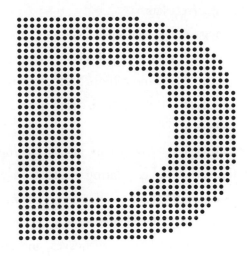

HEALTH AND ENERGY

INFLAMMATION

We tend not to consider inflammation until we encounter an injury or experience pain. In fact, we have varying levels of inflammation occurring at all times. Those who exercise in a high-volume or high-intensity regime will significantly increase their inflammatory response. So what does this have to do with getting your body into shape? Put simply, inflammation causes a decrease in blood flow to and from muscles. This translates into fewer nutrients getting to the muscles and a decreased efficiency in the removal of waste products. Obviously this has quite an impact on your energy, strength, metabolism and overall health. Inflammation is also a major cause of many common diseases. The good news is that you can reduce the inflammatory response through improving your nutrition, in particular eating the correct fats.

Omega-3 and omega-6 fatty acids are 'essential' fats, which means they can't be made from scratch by body cells, nor can the cells convert one to the other. They must be provided by the food we eat. As with any essential nutrient, if we are lacking in these essential fats we will experience ill health.

Essential fatty acids (EFAs) have many important functions. Most notably they act like hormones, regulating blood pressure, blood-clot formation, blood fats, the immune response and inflammation. EFAs also serve as structural parts of cell membranes (outer lining), are a major constituent part of our brain and nerves, and are essential to normal growth and vision in infants and children.

Omega-6 is found in all popular vegetable oils and is generally consumed in excess in our society. While these oils are often touted as healthy, overprocessing and overconsumption can lead to significant health problems. A high consumption of omega-6 can lead to an increase in the production of eicosanoids, which are involved in inflammatory, cardiovascular and immune system diseases. Harmful trans fats are present in overprocessed vegetable oils.

Omega-3 is not as abundant in food as omega-6 is, but it is readily available in oily fish and flaxseed oil (in both fresh and supplement form). Optimum consumption of omega-3 is linked to positive health outcomes, including:

» **decreasing risk for heart disease**

» **decreasing high blood pressure**

» **improving insulin sensitivity for individuals with type 2 diabetes**

>> reducing tenderness in joints in individuals with arthritis

>> assisting with proper development and health of the brain

>> assisting with retina formation for good vision

>> decreasing inflammation

>> protecting against stroke

>> improving cholesterol levels.

Omega-3 and omega-6 are best consumed in a ratio between 1:1 and 1:3 to maximise health benefits. The ratio that exists in modern Western diets ranges from between 1:10 and 1:50. Omega-3 and omega-6 compete for the same enzymes to break them down; because Western diets include such a high level of omega-6, very little omega-3 fat is converted into its active forms of EPA and DHA.

The simple message is to eat cold-water fish, such as salmon and mackerel, two to three times a week and use a high-quality fish oil supplement or cold-pressed flaxseed oil. Normal dosing of these supplements ranges from 3 to 10 grams (3000 mg to 10,000 mg) per day, with each capsule generally 1 gram (1000 mg) in potency. Remember to *always* keep them refrigerated.

ANTIOXIDANTS

Every time you eat, oxygen is required to 'burn' this fuel, providing warmth and energy. Free radicals are a normal by-product of this process. They're also created when you expose yourself to sunlight, ozone, X-rays and radiation, tobacco smoke, fried foods, processed fats and oils, emotional trauma, physical stress, exhaust fumes and the chemical additives in food. I think that includes everything.

There's a war going on inside your body every minute of the day. Under normal circumstances your defence troops (the immune system and antioxidants) can handle the fight, but if you get over stressed or run-down you'll become far more vulnerable to enemy attack. At high levels free radicals can become quite a threat, contributing to the degeneration of our bodies and our health.

The damage, rather than being obviously toxic, is eventually expressed as accelerated ageing or degenerative disease. Free radicals can be controlled within your body at low levels, but if high levels are present they become capable of destruction.

We have all witnessed an apple turning brown after being exposed to oxygen. You can't immediately see the damage being done when you are becoming oxidised but, believe me, many of us are 'turning brown' on the inside.

If free radicals damage your DNA, an eventual consequence could be a higher risk of cancer. If free-radical damage occurs in the arteries that supply blood to your heart, it could eventually lead to a heart attack. Free radicals are now known to be involved in promoting cancer, heart disease, arthritis and perhaps as many as eighty varieties of disease that aren't caused by infection.

For this reason it makes perfect sense to consume antioxidants in your food or as supplements to quench free radicals and minimise potential damage. Antioxidants are the brave soldiers forming your defence troops. They neutralise free radicals and prevent oxidation of fats, thereby safeguarding against excessive damage. Research is still in its infancy, but antioxidants have been shown to prevent or delay many disease processes and to slow degeneration.

The DNA in each cell can be 'hit' as many as 10,000 times a day by free radicals. Unrepaired damage accumulates over a lifetime. This can cause unregulated growth of cells, including tumours and other cell mutations.

So where do we find antioxidants? Colourful plant foods are a great place to start. Some of the most significant antioxidant vitamins are vitamins A, C, E and betacarotene. Minerals such as selenium, zinc and manganese play important roles, as do various enzymes such as coenzyme Q10 and glutathione.

It's recommended that you consume a variety of antioxidants, not just a single one. As with all nutrients, they're most effective when a variety of them are present at one time. Many of us don't get sufficient antioxidant nutrients from our diet. The demand dictated by your body is increasing due to lifestyle changes, as well as chemicals and pollutants in the environment and food processing and storage. Excessive amounts of exercise at higher intensities or in polluted areas will also increase free-radical production in the body.

If you're already consuming an abundance of fresh vegetables, nuts and seeds, you may be covering your requirements. Realistically, I think we could all confess to not consuming adequate quantities of vegetables on a consistent daily basis. My recommendation is to eat around ten servings of plant foods per day, consisting of two servings of fruit and eight of vegetables (one serving is approximately half a cup).

WHEY PROTEIN:
NOT JUST FOR MUSCLE MEN

Whey protein is extracted from whey (the watery part of milk which is separated from curd in the cheesemaking process), which possesses the highest biological value (absorption) of all known forms of protein. The biological value of well-manufactured whey protein isolate (WPI) is 159 — higher than eggs, meat, chicken or any other protein source. Put simply, humans digest and absorb WPI more efficiently than any other protein food.

Not all protein powders are created equal. Many are composed of inferior forms of protein, carefully labelled as 'blends', which sometimes contain as little as 10 per cent desirable proteins. The unfavourable inclusion of additives and fillers essentially dilutes the product purity and, unfortunately, the health benefits. The purest form is microfiltered whey protein isolate (WPI). Containing 90 to 96 per cent protein and no lactose, microfiltered WPI is separated in a way that ensures that micronutrients are not damaged. Other varieties may use harsh chemicals and radiation during this process, denaturing the raw ingredient.

Research has shown whey protein to have a positive effect on stamina, muscle growth, satiety, blood-sugar stability and exercise recovery, as well as accelerating wound healing.

High-quality whey protein provides a rich source of amino acids (building blocks of protein), including glutathione. Glutathione is the body's premier antioxidant and defends cells against free-radical damage, toxins, infection and carcinogens. Low levels of glutathione are associated with many diseases. For active people, low glutathione levels also correlate to poor physical performance. High-quality whey protein increases cell glutathione concentrations, enhances athletic performance and improves body composition.

The amino acid profile of whey protein is most similar to that of human muscle. An optimum supply of the right material promotes better recovery from training and a greater anabolic (preventing muscle wastage) effect. Whey protein is hypo-allergenic, making it suitable for individuals who have allergic reactions or intolerances to other protein supplements.

ESSENTIAL FATS

Mild inflammation occurs in various tissues, such as muscles, connective tissue and joints, after intense physical activity as the immune system becomes engaged in breaking down dead and damaged cells. If this post-exercise inflammatory state becomes too pronounced, healthy cells can also get damaged. Recovery time increases because healthy tissue is also being destroyed by the immune system. Consequently, an exaggerated inflammatory state can occur, largely due to a lack of essential fats.

The primary role of essential fatty acids (EFAs) is energy production, among other functions such as:

» **keeping our cell membranes pliable to enhance nutrient absorption and facilitate the elimination of waste and toxins**

» **shortening recovery time by encouraging cells to better absorb the nutrients needed for recuperation**

» **helping to prevent the damage caused by the consumption of other fats**

» **enhancing the activity of insulin after physical activity.**

Further benefits include antioxidant activity, anti-inflammatory properties, joint health, cardiovascular protection, healthy skin and immune enhancement. A deficiency of EFAs may cause muscle weakness as they're essential for the formation of the healthy fat surrounding muscle tissue.

Intensive exercise causes depletion of EFAs, therefore the more exercise you do, the higher your daily requirement — in extreme cases, up to 20 grams (20,000 mg) per day.

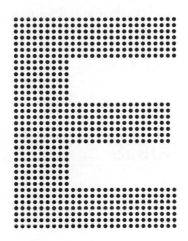

AFTER THE AFTER

One of the most common questions I hear as I near the end of a consultation is, 'So what do I do for maintenance once I reach my goal weight?' The answer is simple, yet often surprises. We've talked about your body being a direct reflection of your lifestyle, and you now know that when you choose your goal weight and follow the modular menu planner you will arrive at your target. Essentially, this too is how you maintain it. You're not eating too few calories, so you won't continue to lose weight beyond your goal weight (I think you'll agree that eternal weight loss hasn't been a major issue for any of us). For example, if you're currently 80 kilos and you choose your goal calorie intake of 70 kilos, your body will plateau once you reach 70 kilos. If you then assume that you can now eat differently, seeing as you no longer need to lose weight, you'll find your weight creeping back up again. Yep, it's that damned mirror image thing again.

The plan simply provides you with exactly what you need to reach and maintain your goal. While it does require some conscious effort to establish your new regime, there are no extreme measures involved in this plan so you shouldn't need to 'go off' it. This plan is sustainable for a lifetime.

EXCUSES, **EXCUSES**

Too busy to exercise? Haven't found time to shop for fresh foods? Too tired to exercise at the end of the working day? It was raining? Your cat died? Yep, I've heard them all.

We know that if we made this many excuses for having days off work, we'd probably lose our jobs. So why not treat our bodies as the best job we'll ever have? Repeat after me: there is no *spare* time, I must *make* time.

Interestingly, if I don't exercise as much as I'd like, I actually lose weight. How does this happen? Well, I adjust my food to match my needs and, if I don't stimulate my muscle, I lose it. Not ideal, I know. But it's better than losing muscle *and* gaining fat simultaneously.

A few of my clients handle holidays quite successfully. If they know they're going away for a few weeks of potential indulgence, they'll work a little harder leading up to their trip to start a couple of kilos down. Effectively they broaden their buffer zone, so at worst they return from their holiday back at their ideal weight.

If you choose — yes, it's a choice now that you've assumed responsibility— to exercise less, even for a period of time, to maintain your weight you must adjust your food intake accordingly. Without the exercise your buffer zone has become much tighter and you have no room for excess. If you'd like your share of excess, you don't have the option of reducing your activity. Simple, huh?

CHANGING YOUR **DEFAULT SETTINGS**

We all seem to have a default setting when it comes to our weight. I know that if I simply relaxed my exercise regime and became just a little careless with my food intake, I'd creep up from my regular 58 kilos to 68 kilos in no time flat. I feel at my best at 58 kilos, so I allow a small buffer zone of 2 kilos each way for maintenance. If I creep up to 60 kilos, I know it's time to up the ante. If I drop to 56 kilos, I realise I've been working too many hours and I need to pay more attention to regular meals. The rule I've set for myself is to *never* stray outside my buffer zone.

When we lose weight we usually need to establish a new buffer zone. If you've been 100 kilos and you're trying to get down to 70 kilos, yet you get stuck at 80 kilos, there are often a few factors at play. Firstly, when everyone has been telling you how fabulously you're doing, whether you acknowledge it or not, a little complacency may have crept in. You're also feeling a lot better in yourself so the urgency of losing further weight begins to fade. You justify the odd binge or lapse in exercise by thinking about the 20 kilos you've lost so far. At this point you're in grave danger of sliding right back to where you started. The first thing you need to do is to change your default and your buffer zone. At my heaviest, I tipped the scales at 85 kilos. This used to be my default. If I kept this in my mind, I could easily justify the scales climbing back up to 70 kilos and still consider myself in better shape than I used to be. Instead, I've narrowed my buffer zone to only 2 kilos each way. Once you have maintained your new buffer zone for a period of time, it will become easier to keep up and the memory of your previous heavier default will fade. Of course, it's much simpler to maintain your goal weight if you reach it by following permanent lifestyle changes rather than an unsustainable quick-fix fad.

Another important thing to remember is not to try to be perfect. To successfully follow a diet plan verbatim you would have to eliminate almost every social event from your calendar and become a hermit. What tends to happen is that we attempt perfection, only to be challenged by normal everyday obstacles such as birthday parties, catered conferences or impromptu dinner invitations. If you allow these occasions to regularly throw you off track you'll narrow your choice to either social isolation or overindulgence. In any situation where you find yourself in less than perfect surroundings just make the best choices possible. If you are at someone's home for dinner, for example, you don't want to be rude and refuse to eat the meal, but nor should you throw caution to the wind and assume that your diet is doomed. Take the middle ground and simply do the best you can to control the portion size of your meal and don't overindulge in the wine and dessert. Moderation is the key. My advice? If a diet and exercise program is too restrictive to follow forever, it's doomed to failure.

BUT WHAT HAPPENS AFTER THE AFTER?

We have seen stars from Oprah Winfrey to Kirstie Alley punch the air in jubilant celebration many times over the years as they shed layers and create new identities, only to watch them seesaw. Fat clothes then skinny clothes; euphoria then depression. You would imagine that these celebrities surround themselves with the best chefs and trainers money can buy, yet they still fall down when it comes to permanent fat loss. Why?

I'm sure there are many reasons, but I have found that when clients don't take full responsibility for their new regime it inevitably fails, regardless of how much cash they throw at it or how substantial their support network is. I have worked with many high-profile clients who will commonly ask me to communicate with their private assistant or their chef to accommodate their lifestyle changes. This may sound like a dream situation to be in, but the minute the client is away from this support network the new regime falls apart. There's a distinct lack of internal knowledge and boundaries, and the individual isn't taking the project seriously enough or assigning it enough priority to handle it themselves. This quickly becomes a very weak link in the fat-loss chain.

As thrilling as it may be to lose weight — and I would be the first to congratulate those who meet their goals — what happens when the high passes, as inevitably it will? You will grow accustomed to your new body, your new image and your new wardrobe.

You need to believe that the rewards of keeping the weight off have to do with much more than your appearance. If you learn to value yourself and your life, taking responsibility for your health is much more enduring than dropping four sizes in your jeans (as gratifying as that may be).

But when the 'new you' gradually becomes commonplace, the praise and attention from others slows and some pitfalls can develop. Remember your journey. Remember the dedication it took to wean yourself off sugar; the friends who mocked you when you left the bread rolls in the basket at your favourite restaurant; the juggling to put aside thirty minutes every day to walk, rain, hail or shine. Remember the first feelings of extra energy and the overall sense of wellbeing that you now take for granted. The new routine took commitment, motivation and dedication. You should be proud of it and honour it by sticking to it. That is the euphoria that lasts a lifetime.

We're all aware of celebrities who have personal trainers, chefs and minders to make getting into shape much easier. And wouldn't we all love to surround ourselves in the same way. But don't forget that these people still have to do the exercise and resist lots of amazingly elaborate food. Just like the rest of us mere mortals, they still do destructive things to their bodies and indulge in fad diets and yo-yo.

Some people think that keeping the weight off is easier for me than for the average person because I work in the fitness industry. But where I work is irrelevant. I stay motivated because, quite simply, I value my life and want to have the best body to live it in.

HYPOTHETICAL #3

THE PROBLEM

Jenny is a twelve-year-old girl who has always struggled with her weight. Her parents are feeling confused and frustrated, not knowing how to help their daughter without putting pressure on her or making her even more self-conscious. She's a fussy eater and does very little exercise. As she gains weight it's increasingly difficult for her to participate in exercise at the same level as her friends. Her parents would like to help her become healthier while she's still young so she avoids a lifetime battle with her weight.

THE SOLUTION

DIET

The focus is on education and health, not weight loss.

» I find a great way to broaden the food choices of a fussy eater is to teach them how to cook. The more Jenny learns about fresh ingredients and their origins, flavours and textures, the more she will develop an interest in healthy foods and perhaps even shy away from highly processed junk food. I'd suggest her parents dust off their recipe books and take Jenny to the market. Better still, help Jenny set up her own little veggie garden.

» Leading by example can have a very strong influence on children of Jenny's age. If the family pantry is filled with healthy, unprocessed foods and everyone is encouraged to eat primarily fresh foods, this will become second nature. Much of our palate and our relationship with food is formed throughout our childhood, so poor habits can be difficult to change in adulthood.

» It's important to set boundaries for Jenny to avoid poor food choices. She needs to recognise that some foods are treats that we can only have on special occasions, while others are everyday foods. Portion control is another important factor. Once Jenny is consuming fresh, unprocessed foods, this will likely regulate her appetite and help to minimise the cravings for sugar and treats.

» I'd suggest getting Jenny involved in packing her lunchbox with healthy alternatives, perhaps even snacks she's helped to make herself. School canteens can have many unhealthy temptations for children, so packing her lunch for at least four days a week will help remove some of these foods from her day.

» Jenny's parents can organise to have some healthy snacks awaiting her when she arrives home from school, such as fresh fruit, veggie sticks and a homemade low-cal dip, cherry tomatoes or perhaps a Ryvita crispbread with cheese and tomato.

STRENGTH

It's important, even at Jenny's age, to stay strong.

» Sometimes children don't have the attention span to exercise in a gym environment, so I'd suggest getting Jenny involved in a team sport, or perhaps a class at the local health club, such as boxercise, gymnastics, rock-climbing or dance. Anything that gets her moving and incorporates some element of strength would be brilliant.

» The local park will likely have a playground with a variety of monkey bars and climbing equipment which will improve strength and coordination.

CARDIO

Thirty to sixty minutes a day.

» Cardio needn't feel like 'exercise' to children (or adults, for that matter). Jenny can ride her bike to and from school, play ball in the park with friends or go for a walk after school with her mum or dad. All of these activities are both highly effective and fun.

» There are many enjoyable activities Jenny can do from home on her own or with friends and family, such as rollerblading, hitting a tennis ball against a wall, shooting hoops, playing hopscotch, skipping or even Wii Fit.

CONCLUSION

MEDICAL MADNESS

As we increasingly turn to doctors as obesity specialists, we should be aware that in the many years of training to become a GP, nutrition, health and exercise play a very insignificant part. I train and advise several doctors who all readily attest to this.

Growing numbers of people visit their doctor searching for weight loss and dietary advice. The obesity epidemic has become a highly lucrative industry and the obese are vulnerable targets. Medical 'obesity specialists' are sometimes quick to recommend extreme measures which can lead to chronic conditions in years to come.

Looking externally for the answer is always easier than facing the fact that you are the key to a healthier, happier life. While it's wise to see a physician to evaluate your general state of health, be diligent with your homework about obesity specialists. Ask about their training, their level of education and what advice criteria they work from. Better still, do your own research to find the approach that suits your lifestyle. While experts in a specific field — ranging from surgery to disease diagnosis and pharmaceutical prescription — all play a significant role in the treatment of disease, many are dishing out advice despite knowing very little about nutrition, exercise, general health, lifestyle habits and the physical or psychological reasons behind excessive weight gain.

Clearly we aren't overfat because our stomachs are the wrong size or because we have excess intestine, yet surgical intervention to 'correct' these issues reigns supreme. There are two common forms of bariatric surgery: lap (gastric) band and gastric bypass. A lap band makes the stomach smaller to enforce smaller meals. As the name suggests, gastric bypass surgery bypasses a section of intestine where we absorb much of our calorie intake. We also absorb our essential nutrients in this way, so we're missing out on a lot more than just excess calories, and nutritional deficiencies and related ailments are likely to result.

A lap band is generally a fluid-filled band placed around the stomach to reduce its capacity. The fluid levels can then be altered to reduce or increase capacity as required. To date I have met fourteen recipients of this surgery, and I have yet to see a result that could be considered truly 'successful'.

While lap bands are generally reserved for the obese, one woman I've worked with was only 20 kilos over her ideal weight. On examination of her diet twelve weeks after surgery, I found that her capacity to consume food was at less than 50 per cent of her minimum metabolic requirement. This, combined with her lack of knowledge of nutrition, meant that her nutritional intake was extremely deficient. When I suggested that she return to her specialist to discuss whether he should remove some fluid from the band to allow her to consume adequate nutrition, she said she was frightened to have any fluid removed in case she stopped losing weight. In this case, the lap band was clearly perpetuating an already unhealthy attitude towards food and the patient's body image, which raises questions for me about the profiling for suitability carried out prior to such surgery (besides bank balance, that is). The band had become a crutch on which she felt completely reliant in order to stay on track. Her nutrition was poor, her education about eating healthily hadn't improved, the psychological reasons for her previous bingeing weren't being addressed or resolved and she was losing a significant amount of her 'weight' in lean muscle tissue, which is necessary to maintain a normal metabolism. This is a dangerous (and common) downhill spiral: easy to enter and very difficult to recover from.

I have heard many surgeons profess that this type of surgery is only considered an option when all other weight-loss methods fail. Perhaps they are failing because of the multitude of unsustainable fads? Perhaps overweight individuals require further common-sense education about diet and exercise, often in conjunction with some form of psychological therapy to overcome compulsive eating patterns and destructive behaviour. While weight-loss surgery may provide a short-term band-aid solution, these outstanding issues cannot be surgically removed.

Do your research on the health professional from whom you intend to seek help and guidance. Remember, if you ask the advice of a surgeon, it's likely that the solution will be surgery.

While lap-band surgeries are becoming an increasingly popular weight-loss 'solution' across the globe, some disturbing statistics are emerging. A staggering 15 per cent of these surgeries fail, resulting in a second operation to reverse or revise the procedure. Considering the dangers of general anaesthesia and major surgery for obese individuals, the high likelihood of a second anaesthetic alone poses a genuine risk to life. Some would argue that lap-band candidates are risking their lives if they don't elect for surgery, but as with any such intervention, there are very real risks involved.

Over an eight-year period (2000 to 2008) the NHS saw 6953 obesity surgeries, with laparoscopic adjustable gastric banding

(LAGB) being the most popular method used throughout Europe. In 2010, this number had grown to around 12,000–14,000 surgeries per annum, of which approximately 8000–10,000 were in the private sector. Around 350,000 bariatric surgeries are performed worldwide each year, 63 per cent of which take place in the USA. Researchers from the University of California, San Diego, have reported that a significant number of these surgeries are unsuccessful, with 15–20 per cent of gastric bypass patients regaining much of their weight within a few years following the procedure. As a nation, the UK saw a 55 per cent rise in these surgeries during 2009, costing in the region of £20 million. Professor Tony Leeds of Whittington Hospital in North London warns that an estimated one million Britons qualify to receive this surgery on the NHS, which could potentially cost £9.1 billion.

Dr John Jorgensen, a gastrointestinal surgeon, said redoing lap bands was becoming 'a disease in itself'. 'The ridiculous thing is that after a band fails, surgeons just tend to put a new one in,' Dr Jorgensen said. 'Isn't that the definition of insanity?'

My sentiments exactly.

STOP THE INSANITY ...

Over the past twenty years I thought I'd seen and heard almost every radical method of weight loss. Little did I know that the most preposterous was yet to come: the possibility of bariatric surgery for children.

The option of surgical treatment for obesity is becoming all too common. Doctors often promote this as a last resort to combat the 'disease' that is obesity, and yet these radical procedures are being made available to our children.

It sounds like the magic answer: you can shed kilos and get 'healthy' without having to do a thing. No willpower, no education about food choices, no gruelling exercise regime. It's the light at the end of a long tunnel of yo-yo diets, low self-esteem and the burden of carrying around those extra kilos. All it takes is for your child to undergo a general anaesthetic for a major surgical procedure that distorts their stomach to ensure they can only consume a restrictive, nutritionally poor food intake. The subsequent malnutrition would no doubt cause a multitude of ailments for an adult, let alone the developing body of a child.

The problem not being addressed is that obesity is not a disease. Our children are not overweight due to a lap-band deficiency, nor were they born with a deformed, oversized stomach. Sure, there are some genetic influences, but there are also myriad lifestyle choices associated with all cases of obesity. It often runs in families because the family unit has created and perpetuated poor lifestyle habits. I acknowledge that becoming obese is rarely intentional, but the thousands of obese men, women and teenagers I have helped over the years are generally misinformed and require a full education on healthy lifestyle habits — not a scalpel. This sensible and effective approach not only reduces the risk of serious health issues surrounding obesity, but it teaches the individual how to maintain a healthy body, which in turn will be passed on through future generations. This is the only long-term solution to the obesity epidemic, not surgical intervention.

Obesity is not a disease but a symptom. It's not bacterial or viral. It may be considered a disease of lifestyle and it may cause disease, but it's self-imposed and reversible. Surgery, on the other hand, is a lot more complicated. People who have lap-band surgery are restricted to a diet of processed foods because they can't digest 'real' fibrous foods, such as fresh, colourful plant foods, unless they are puréed to mush. Lap-band patients who have attempted to eat 'real' wholefoods have vividly described to me the resulting projectile vomit. One woman had resorted to eating children's biscuits for dinner because they were soft enough for her to digest and didn't cause discomfort or regurgitation. She had lost a few kilos, but her hair was falling out by the handful.

The common medical advice given to lap-band patients after surgery is to exercise and watch what they eat. Why can't we encourage and educate our children to follow this advice without the risk of anaesthetic and major surgery, leading to a lifetime of restriction? Surgical intervention leads to a range of health problems. Apart from the inherent dangers they face from a diet of highly processed foods, such patients also find it difficult to digest fats, further excluding the benefits of omega-3 fatty acids, which help protect the vascular and skeletal systems and facilitate normal brain function.

We want to believe that obesity is a disease that has somehow been imposed on us. Whether the perceived 'cure' is lap-band surgery or a miraculous new pill or potion, there's no magic bullet or surgeon's knife that will solve the obesity epidemic among our children. Until we take responsibility for our damaging lifestyle choices, it is not possible for us to find the way into the light of health and appropriate body composition. Reality television shows only perpetuate the belief that extreme exercise, pain, sweat and tears are the only other solutions. No wonder so many are swayed towards the knife. Fortunately, there is a highly effective happy medium that is easy to follow with a bit of guidance and knowledge.

I strongly urge greater in-school education for parents and children about food choices, exercise and general lifestyle before we create a malnourished generation with a new epidemic of associated health risks.

THE FUTURE OF FAT LOSS

In recent years obesity costs have escalated, with the figures now into the billions every year. In addition to the government subsidies that overweight and obese people might receive, including payments for disability, mobility and sickness allowances, and unemployment benefits, there are direct healthcare costs — ambulatory services, hospitalisation, prescription medication and some medically related consumables, such as blood-glucose self-monitoring meters and strips — and direct non-healthcare costs such as transport to hospital, supported accommodation and special foods.

Since I joined the health and fitness industry I have witnessed the evolution of an empire. 'Experts' dish out conflicting and confusing diet information — in very large portions. In fact, if we did what all the experts told us, we'd do more of everything while doing less of everything. We'd exercise earlier, later and not at all. Fat would make us healthy and kill us, carbs would make us thin and fat and protein would turn us into gods and goddesses and put us on dialysis.

There is one fundamental fact that no-one can refute. We need to move and eat a healthy diet to shed kilos.

These days our lives are becoming increasingly sedentary and, with our waistlines expanding, exercise is no longer a luxury but a necessity. Personal trainers used to be a status symbol, a bit like mobile phones once were — only for the rich and famous. Yet despite this shift we are still getting fatter. While exercise is a very important factor in fat loss and health, it's rarely successful in the absence of dietary changes. One of the most common excuses for inactivity and weight gain is lack of time. Many of us spend our days at work exhausting our minds but not our bodies. All the while, we consume convenience foods that are calorie-rich and nutrient-poor.

THE FITNESS **REVOLUTION**

I managed to make it through the aerobics-obsessed, Lycra-clad phase of the 1980s, but many Baby Boomers are still living with aching, mangled joints as a result of those high-impact classes. Exercise has since progressed to more ergonomic and lower-impact weight training, Pilates, yoga and elliptical machines. The popularity of 'smart' or 'functional' training, using focused core and dynamic training methods, is a growing trend for the better.

Technology is now able to compare our chronological age (time) with our biological age (state of health). Alarmingly, many thirty-year-olds are walking around in fifty-year-old bodies! From complete blood profiles to the physical testing of individuals, we can determine the rate of damage accrued through such factors as lifestyle choices, diet and stress levels. The great news is that with the right lifestyle changes it is possible to turn back the clock.

Teaching individuals to manage time by incorporating more movement into daily routines is one of the keys to a healthy future. Instead of sitting down to read, catch up on world news or even watch a movie, do it on an exercise machine or listen while walking. While advances in technology are often blamed for making us more sedentary, they have also provided the luxury of being able to download content and move as you watch, read or listen.

We are becoming more educated about the importance of body composition as opposed to weight on the scales. From body composition apparatus to software programs, more sophisticated devices are being developed to measure our progress and set up realistic goals to achieve long-term results. One example of this is my own professional-use software, Aston Rx, which is used to determine individual body composition and goal structure, and to produce a week-by-week timeline to achieve the goals. A precise calorie requirement is then converted into a diet planner specific to the individual.

Research efforts have shifted our focus to the health benefits of dietary improvements and the development of new foods as well as a greater understanding of existing ones.

Functional foods that prevent the early onset of ageing and disease, dubbed 'nutraceuticals', are being developed. As the combination of the words 'nutrition' and 'pharmaceutical' suggests, nutraceuticals are foods or food products that provide health and medical benefits, including having a role in the prevention and treatment of disease.

All vegetables are good but some are more beneficial than others. An increasing number of so-called 'superfoods' are now recognised for their superior nutritional content and their ability to keep us looking and feeling at our best. These include some old faithfuls, such as blueberries and cruciferous vegetables (which include broccoli, cabbage and Brussels sprouts). There's no scientific definition of a superfood; this is an informal category of foods that are particularly high in health benefits. In a contest between iceberg lettuce and spinach, for instance, spinach would be the victor. Both vegetables have vitamin C and fibre, but spinach also offers folate and antioxidants such as lutein and zeaxanthin, which may help prevent vision loss from macular degeneration as we age.

Some innovations are a bit of fun, but aren't necessarily going to encourage couch potatoes to get up and move. The sporting apparel giants have developed shoes linked to our iPods to show us the distance we've travelled, while GPS technology (once reserved for navigating our cars) is being used to track and motivate runners worldwide. Some companies have computerised their running shoes to adapt to our individual running styles and determine the strike patterns of our feet as we run, reacting with cushioning where it's most needed. A clever idea, but probably more suited for the serious trainer.

DIET AND **FITNESS MYTHS**

Several years ago I was invited to Switzerland by a keen triathlete who was seeking advice on how to improve her diet, achieve her endurance goals and lose a few kilos of body fat to enhance her speed and overall performance. Kerry had been training for and competing in triathlons for several years, but was frustrated at having reached a plateau. She had sought the advice of numerous dieticians and coaches in previous months, all to no avail. Kerry had recently observed the appearance of some cellulite on the back of her thighs; when she mentioned this the team dietician had promptly asked if Kerry ate cottage cheese. Although this seemed like an odd question, Kerry answered, 'Yes, regularly. Why?' The dietician proclaimed: 'If you eat cottage cheese then your thighs will begin to look like cottage cheese.' Yes, I'm afraid she was serious. Heaven knows what happens when we eat jelly!

MYTH:

Specific exercises will tone up fat.

FACT:

The state of our flabby upper arms, pot tummy or any other unwelcome bulges is determined by our body composition — the ratio of lean muscle to stored body fat. To improve the condition of specific body parts you must first make changes to your overall body composition by increasing lean muscle and decreasing stored fat. You can develop great muscle tone by targeting specific body parts with various exercises, but until you make the necessary lifestyle changes to reduce the body fat it's hiding beneath, you'll never know it's there. To achieve tone and definition, dietary modifications combined with fat-burning cardiovascular exercise and resistance training are essential. It sounds a little daunting, I know, but that's why I've written two user-friendly books to help you on your way.

Most people don't distinguish between muscle and stored fat, harbouring unrealistic expectations of somehow making the stored fat transform itself into shapely, firm muscle. This is a physical impossibility that will result in failure and disappointment every time.

MYTH:
There is no 'cure' for cellulite.

FACT:
Rubbish! While cellulite is not some dreaded disease requiring a 'cure', it can be eliminated. Marketing gurus have tried to pin the blame on everything from 'toxic build-up' to 'trapped fat'   and, of course, they have the quick fix. One recent advertisement claimed to sell a cream that would 'liquidise congested cellulite and pass it into our lymphatic system for excretion'. That's like saying that if you rub a cream on your car bonnet, the petrol will make its way through the engine and evaporate.

Let's clear this one up once and for all. You may have noticed that men rarely have cellulite. Women's hormones dictate our distribution of body fat. Our wonderful child-bearing bodies tend to store a little reserve of extra fat cells around the hips and thighs, and when filled with fat they often result in rather unfortunate lumps and bumps. This is subcutaneous fat, which means that it lies just beneath the skin.

Fat cells are like balloons that can be inflated when they're required to store excess energy as body fat. The number of fat cells is fixed in adulthood, but each fat cell is capable of great expansion. The amount of excess energy we consume (or how much we burn) is the primary dictator of the amount of body fat stored at any one time. When an excess of fat beyond a certain density is stored beneath the skin, the visible accumulation of an uneven distribution results in what we know as cellulite.

In a nutshell: cellulite is a fancy name for an excess of stored subcutaneous body fat concentrated in a specific area. Call it any name you like, but if you store an overall excess of body fat, the dimpled appearance will be more pronounced.

The good news? By modifying your lifestyle and consequently reducing your overall stored body fat, you can banish cellulite. And save your money — no lotions, pills or potions can do this for you.

MYTH:
Our body fat is genetically determined and cannot be altered.

FACT:

The quantity and distribution of fat storage cells may be influenced by genetics, lifestyle choices and hormones, but whether you choose to fill them up with excess stored energy is completely up to you — not your genes. For example, if your family has a history of big thighs, this doesn't have to be your destiny. If you do gain excess weight, there's a good chance that it will be in these predetermined areas. It's your own lifestyle that will influence whether or not you fill these storage tanks. Blaming it on Great Auntie June just doesn't cut it.

MYTH:

Eating carbs after 4 pm will cause weight gain.

FACT:

If a food is good for you in the morning, it is not going to be bad for you after some mystical hour of the afternoon. This is yet another deceitful way of imposing calorie (or carbohydrate) restrictions.

Carbohydrates are not all created equal. Avoiding all processed carbohydrate foods, such as white flour products, processed commercial cereals, biscuits, pastries and sugars, should be a twenty-four-hour deal. Weight loss aside, these products are not good for our health and supply us with nutritionally empty calories, no matter what the time of day. It's preferable to stick with the vast choice of whole, unprocessed carbohydrates. You'll be pleased to know that you don't even have to glance at your watch.

MYTH:

Liposuction is the only way to successfully remove that stubborn fat that can't be shifted with diet and exercise. Once surgically removed, the fat will never come back.

FACT:

There's no such thing as excess body fat that can't be removed without the help of surgery. Believe me, I lost my own 'saddle bags' without resorting to liposuction. I'm not going to lie to you, it's tough work. And it's the first place it all comes back if I allow myself to gain a little fat.

I often hear people say that they've tried everything and nothing seems to work. I have even heard this from medical professionals. Do you think it was a coincidence that they were surgeons specialising in liposuction? It's what we all want to hear: it's not our fault and we can't fix it no matter how hard we try, so the surgeons will fix it for us.

The fact is that we store excess body fat as an energy reserve. Once you allow your body to use this stored energy, the fat will come off (as long as your goals are realistic). I don't doubt that disillusioned dieters have tried various methods of fat loss, but that doesn't mean that nothing will work.

As for fat never returning after surgery — the fat cells that are removed do not make their way back to you, but the many cells that remain have an amazing ability to expand beyond our wildest dreams. If your lifestyle before liposuction encouraged fat storage, it is unlikely that you will change to an appropriate post-surgery diet to maintain any fat loss. If this were the case, you could have done this initially and eliminated the need for the surgery in the first place. In fact, many people think that they can go wild on food after liposuction in the belief that the fat cannot return. I vividly recall a friend proudly announcing that she had just had 2 kilos of fat removed by liposuction. In the following five weeks she had to wear post-surgical bandaging and was advised not to exert herself. During this sedentary period she gained 7 kilos. You do the maths!

SIX COMMON FAT-LOSS MISTAKES

It should be working. You've followed your chosen plan to the letter. You've clocked up enough treadmill kilometres to get you to Timbuktu and back, yet that extra padding is clinging on to your thighs for dear life. Surely by now you should be enjoying the fruits of your labour. So what could you possibly be doing wrong?

Before frustration sets in and you dive headfirst into the next fad diet, let's assess the fundamental flaws that can halt the majority of our dieting efforts and, most importantly, those elusive results.

#1

THE NEED FOR SPEED

I can't stress enough the importance of setting realistic goals. Not only should they be appropriate for your body, but also for your lifestyle and your schedule. The need to diet often begins when we reach a point of despair with our current body shape. Of course at this stage we all want results yesterday, hence the common overly drastic, quick-fix approach.

It's a good idea to calculate exactly how much body fat you need to lose. Rather than looking at the often-daunting 'big picture', you can then establish a realistic timeline to reach your goal. This will not only provide you with direction, but may also help to sustain motivation and act as a positive reinforcement each time you achieve the stepping stones along the way.

#2
THE YO-YO STRATEGY

Sometimes we trust an old strategy because it worked once before. My question is: if it was so effective, why did you stop? To be truly successful, changes in your diet must be implemented for life — not just for a couple of weeks to lose a few kilos. If you feel you must revert back to 'normal', your strategy is likely the wrong one for you.

In my experience, long-term strategies are usually developed over time. It's not a case of simply following in the dietary footsteps of your favourite Hollywood star. A successful strategy involves you listening to your body, gathering information and forging new habits that fit into your own daily life, without forcing you to turn everything upside down to accommodate your regime.

#3
OVERDOING IT

One of the most common fat-loss mistakes is eating too few calories and doing too much exercise. Besides making you feel awful and raising your risk of injury and illness, starvation of nutrition and calories combined with overexertion is dangerous. There's no use trying to compensate for a poor diet by exercising to the extreme. You may think that you're getting away with it and, from a calorie point of view, you just might be. However, it will play havoc with your health and metabolism in the long term.

By restricting your calories below the amount you require to maintain your healthy body weight you risk losing muscle, sending your metabolic rate into a nose dive. While you may see a temporary loss of weight on the bathroom scales, a sluggish metabolism will make your quest for fat loss increasingly difficult and almost impossible to maintain.

#4
IT'S ALL TOO MUCH

Although it's difficult to overeat good, wholesome foods, it is possible. Calories are energy that must be burned. Serial dieters are often so accustomed to deprivation that when they give themselves permission to eat a particular food, they tend to go overboard.

We're usually at low risk of overeating foods in their unprocessed state. As nature intended, unprocessed carbohydrates, lean protein and 'friendly' fats help to switch on feelings of satiety and prevent overconsumption of calories. Just be wary of hidden additives in commercial 'health foods'. Read labels carefully: many diet foods contain numerous sugars, sweeteners and thickeners, bumping up the calories and increasing the likelihood of fat gain.

#5
THE ROLLER-COASTER

In recent years it's become more widely accepted that sugar-laden foods have a significant effect on our blood-sugar levels, are detrimental to health and are largely accountable for much of the population's excess body fat.

Controlling your blood-sugar levels by avoiding sugary foods and beverages and consuming wholefoods, friendly fats (as found in fish, avocado and nuts) and lean protein not only elevates your energy, mood and concentration, but also encourages optimum fat loss and keeps your sweet tooth at bay. Diets high in processed carbohydrates and sugars can exacerbate cravings and overeating, making fat loss close to impossible.

#6
INACCURATE FEEDBACK

Just because the bathroom scales are not showing a significant loss in overall weight doesn't necessarily mean that your efforts have been in vain. If you're gaining lean muscle through exercise while losing fat, your overall weight loss may appear slow on the scales. For example, if you gained 1 kilo of muscle and lost 1 kilo of fat, your weight would remain the same yet your appearance, tone, shape and size would be showing positive changes.

Don't use the scales as your only method of measuring your progress. Acknowledge changes in the way your clothes fit, as well as changes in your overall body shape, tone and strength. If you don't trust your own judgement, it might be a good idea to have your body composition measured and professionally monitored to accurately reflect your progress.

Just remember, if you continue to follow the same strategy, you will get the same results. Perhaps it's time to rethink your body-shaping plan and adopt a few modifications to kickstart some positive change.

INDEX

ACKNOWLEDGEMENTS

What a pleasure it has been working with the Hardie Grant team. Fran Berry — thank you for having confidence in my work. My editor, Rose, what can I say ... patient, passionate and professional. A super talent at your craft. Thank you for putting up with me and my often peculiar ways! My long-time buddy Linda Roach — your wisdom and advice are priceless. Ken Pryor and Tony Reynolds — thanks again for your combined genius. A big thank you to my loyal clients and readers for being such an inspiration and to my brilliant Aston Fitness team for helping to free up my time enough to start writing again. I'm very grateful to all of my friends and colleagues who have contributed testimonials and quotes in this book. Dr Mei Ling Doery — you were the one who gave me that extra nudge to start writing. Thank you for the inspiration and your compelling foreword. Finally, to my husband, David ... always supportive of all I do. Thank you!